Heart to Heart

HEART
to
HEART

A Personal Plan for Creating a Heart-Healthy Family:
Your Guide to the Good Life

Lori Mosca, MD, PhD
Foreword by Mehmet OZ, MD

Health Communications, Inc.
Deerfield Beach, Florida

www.bcibooks.com

Library of Congress Cataloging-in-Publication Data

Mosca, Lori.
 Heart to heart : a personal plan for creating a heart-healthy family your
guide to the good life / Lori Mosca ; foreword by Mehmet Oz.
  p. cm.
 ISBN 0-7573-0245-9
 1. Coronary heart disease—Prevention—Popular works. I. Title.

RC685.C6.M675 2005
616.1'2305—dc22

                2005047181

©2005 Lori Mosca
ISBN 0-7573-0245-9

HCI, its Logos and Marks are trademarks of Health Communications, Inc.

Publisher: Health Communications, Inc.
     3201 S.W. 15th Street
     Deerfield Beach, FL 33442-8190

Cover design by Andrea Perrine Brower
Inside book design by Dawn Von Strolley Grove

For my father—

my first patient and my inspiration.

Contents

Contents

Chapter 9

Chapter 10

Appendix

Foreword

Heart health is a serious matter. But that doesn't mean it has to be a bore. Too often we think of doctor visits as nothing more than needle pricks, weigh-ins and confusing tests. The doctor listens to our problems for five minutes then prescribes a bunch of drugs that our insurance may not even cover. We leave confused and frustrated—and with the clear impression that health is not only beyond our ability to comprehend, but simply too much work to achieve.

There's a revolutionary view of health being championed today, and that is the Dr. Lori Mosca family-based approach. She believes you are the cog in the center of the wheel. The spokes are your loved ones, and together you move forward toward a healthy and fulfilling future.

Families don't just share memories and special occaisions. They also share genes and lifestyles that might put them at risk for heart disease. At our hospital, Dr. Mosca has built a program to help the family members of the cardiac patients I operate on learn about their own risk, so they don't end up in the hospital, too. That's right; she tries to put me out of business! While I operate on diseased hearts, Dr. Mosca asks, "Why wait? Why not save your heart now, before a crisis? Why take the chance that it's going to be too late?"

Dr. Mosca is one of the leading experts in the world in heart disease prevention, and I have no doubt that her revolutionary plan for keeping reluctant patients (she calls them people) healthy has saved thousands of lives. Her approach is practical, it's specific, but it's not strict. It's not a task you give yourself to accomplish; it's a gift you give yourself to enjoy. In this amazing book, *Heart to Heart*, she gives you the blueprint for health that she has spent twenty years of hard work perfecting. And unlike other plans, it's not 50 percent perspiration and 50 percent self-denial, but 100 percent pure joy in the pleasures of life.

In this book, you're also going to meet a truly remarkable person. Dr. Mosca opens up her life to show you the personal side of heart health—from her emotional struggle to deal with her father's heart attack to the triathlons and athletics she participates in with her husband, Ralph, a pediatric cardiac surgeon, and their two sons, Mike and Matt. She shares her patients' personal feelings, their challenges and their successes at walking the talk. This book is filled with the warmth that fuels Dr. Mosca's personal passion for health. She truly cares for each of her patients, and in these pages it shows.

I've known Lori Mosca for more than fifteen years, since we were both in training at Columbia University Medical Center, and I know that she practices what she teaches. Even more important, from a personal and even a health standpoint, she cherishes her family and friends. She understands the importance of setting priorities, of never letting your life get away from you. Dr. Lori Mosca is an inspiration to us all. She shows that you can be at the top of your profession and still be home to cook your son a meal before picking him up from swim practice. And you can be happy.

Let me say that again, because I believe, like Dr. Mosca, that it is essential to your overall health and quality of life. You don't have to feel stressed out, stretched thin and guilty about the things you could have or should have done. You can be calm, confident and happy. And when you are happy, you will be healthy. And when you are healthy, the rest of your family will be healthy, too. It happens in just that order and just that way. It won't happen overnight; after all, habits are hard to break. But it will happen.

Dr. Mosca's goal, ever since I've known her, is to make the world a healthier place that we will all benefit from—and to have a great time doing it! She has already succeeded in helping so many of my patients and countless others. Now let her help you and your family.

—*Mehmet Oz, MD*

Acknowledgments

I wrote a proposal for a book called *Heart to Heart* almost ten years ago, and if it weren't for the persistence and encouragement of Bret Witter, editorial director at Health Communications, Inc., it might still be an idea rather than a reality. Bret convinced me not only to share inspiring patient stories but also to discuss my personal experiences in overcoming barriers to heart disease prevention. It took a lot of nudging, but I think in the end it proved a unique way to reach out to busy people, just like me, who are trying to make better lives for themselves and their families.

As fate would have it, a bicycle accident while training for a triathlon created an opportunity for me to start the book. I could not move my arm for some time, so I enlisted the writing and editorial assistance of Sandra Gordon. She came to my house (I could not drive for a few months), so I could dictate the first draft of *Heart to Heart*. I could not have found another person who made me feel more comfortable sharing my personal and professional journey. She transcribed my words into a seamless story and through her questions assisted me in understanding what would be most helpful and appealing to readers. I was lucky that I did not suffer permanent damage from the accident, but even luckier that I found Sandra. I can't thank her enough for all her support, flexibility and professionalism.

They say the devil is in the details, and it is no different when writing a book or pursuing a career. The full-time, professional staff I work with on a day-to-day basis at NewYork-Presbyterian Hospital and Columbia University, and who allow me to thrive, includes Lisa Rehm, B.S., Heidi Mochari, R.D., M.P.H., Allison Linfante, Ed.D., Dana Edelman, M.P.H., and Karen Ochoa, B.S. They are the wind beneath my wings and make it a pleasure and a privilege to be in the field of preventive cardiology. I want to thank each of them for their helpful comments on the book and their contributions to patient education materials over the years, much of which has been incorporated into *Heart to Heart*. Our team has always looked for creative and engaging ways to disseminate information about heart disease prevention to the public, and I greatly appreciate all they have done for me personally as well as for the greater good.

This is a book about family, and I am fortunate in life to have an extensive one. An academic career in medicine is not easy, and it often requires a lot of travel. I wish to thank all my colleagues, who I consider my extended family, who have sat at the same table and taught me, challenged me, laughed with me and occasionally cried with me. It has made all the sacrifices seem like a blessing. There are also numerous students, residents and fellows who I mentored over the years but who really served as my teachers, and I thank them for inspiring me to carry on. I could not have gone the distance without the support of my mother, Sonya LaBella, who at a moment's notice would drop everything and come watch my kids so I could travel and build my career. While my father, Joseph LaBella, provided vital moral support, Mom was really the one who made all things possible for me to accomplish. My husband of more than twenty years, Ralph Mosca, has supported me through all the bumps in the road of a medical career and has been an amazing father as well as an extraordinary doctor himself. Our two sons, Matt and Mike, provide the meaning and fun behind everything we do, and I thank them for letting me share their lives and dreams. It is because my family lives *Heart to Heart* that it became a book.

Chapter

1

The Wake-Up Call

*"Nothing in life is to be feared,
only to be understood."*

—Marie Curie

"I feel like I have a vice on my chest."

I'll never forget those words from my very first "patient." It was 1982, and I was twenty-three, a second-year medical student studying for the medical boards in the wee hours of a morning in May. Until that point in my career, medicine was confined to lectures and textbooks. But then came the 2 A.M. knock, knock at my door—and the wake-up call that would change my life forever. It was my dad.

"Dad? Dad, what's the matter?"

If I ever saw a heart attack, this is it, I remember thinking when I saw my father, Joe LaBella, a fifty-three-year-old mail carrier from Syracuse, New York, bracing himself against the threshold of my childhood bedroom. It was like something you might now see in a movie or a television commercial for a heart disease drug: Dad's fist was clenched to his heart, his T-shirt dampened in a stripe right down the middle. Clearly, Dad was in trouble, but at least he didn't have to go far to look for help. To keep expenses down throughout medical school, I lived at home. Dad simply had to lumber up a flight of stairs. Still, what I offered in terms of convenience, I lacked in experience. Dad was probably having a heart attack. That much I knew. But what to do?

Call an ambulance? As it turns out, that wasn't an option. A proud Italian male, my father insisted that I *not* lift the phone—that we quietly slip out of the house to a local emergency room. "Don't tell your mother, and don't call the rescue squad, because it will wake her," he instructed, refuting my plan. That was just like Dad, not wanting to bother or worry anyone. He never wanted to let on if he was having a problem. Still, the fact he came to me for help clued me in. *This must be really bad.* I thought for a second. *If I insist on phoning for help anyway, Dad will probably worry so much about upsetting Mom that he'll have an even worse heart attack and drop dead.* I reasoned that I had been a lifeguard for ten years by then, so I knew CPR. I could help him if he had a problem. So that was that. We got in the car and headed to the emergency room.

CPR—An Important Skill

When the heart stops completely during an attack (cardiac arrest), and the person loses consciousness and stops breathing, cardiopulmonary resuscitation (CPR) can save lives. I remember clearly one patient whose life was saved because his wife knew and performed CPR. It's an important skill to know that can help you be prepared in the event of a heart attack or another life-threatening situation. To locate a CPR training center near you, log on to the American Heart Association Web site at *www.americanheart.org* and check under the "Find a Class" option.

On our clandestine mission, Dad and I drove down Woodbine Avenue, past the rows of small but well-kept single- and double-family homes. They were filled with the children, parents and grandparents we knew, people who shared everything from driveways to major life experiences. We moved to the Syracuse neighborhood after our family of seven outgrew a flat in the inner city. As I'd done a thousand times since I was old enough to drive, I stopped at the intersection, waiting to turn left onto James Street, which would take us to the hospital. In the middle of the night, the streets were eerily empty. Still, I dutifully waited at the red light for what seemed like hours. Fortunately, Dad had his senses. "Go through the light, Lori," he said gently, peering into my eyes. It was then it hit me. *Dad's really having a heart attack. He might die.* The fear welled up. I pressed on the accelerator.

You can probably imagine the doctors, nurses and orderlies running around in the emergency room, putting IVs in Dad, just trying to do all this *stuff.* I told the attending physician I was a medical student and pretty sure my father was having a heart attack. When the emergency room physician showed me the results of Dad's electrocardiogram (ECG), which is the most important initial diagnostic test to be administered when a heart attack is suspected, I pretended I could read it, but my mind was spinning. "Your father is having a heart attack, and I need you to make a decision," she said. I was filled with dread. Making a life-or-death call was the last thing I wanted to do in that already stress-filled moment. In fact, what began running through my mind like a ticker tape was not, *What can we do to treat Dad?* but *What could we have done to prevent this?*

As it turns out, the hospital was participating in one of the early pharmaceutical clinical studies of thrombolytic therapy, testing what we now call "clot-busting" drugs, which are used to dissolve blood clots blocking an artery during a heart attack. We now know that clot busters open up the artery and restore blood flow to the heart. They're crucial for stopping a heart attack in its tracks. To be most effective, they need to be administered as soon as possible after symptoms begin.

But at that point in medical history, we were still finding our way. Folks in the throes of a heart attack like Dad would be needed to help researchers make that determination. Did I want Dad to participate in the clot-buster study? I yearned to call my mother, who was still at home, asleep, to get her input, but there wasn't time. "You need to decide right now," the physician said.

I took a minute to explain the situation to my father, who was by this time rigged to an arsenal of equipment, an unnerving beep . . . beep . . . beep in the background. Maybe he would know what to do. Don't dads know everything? "You decide," he said. My twenty-three-year-old mind ran through the options. If Dad received the new drug, there was some risk of internal bleeding, which wasn't good. But there was also a chance that the damage his heart endured from the heart attack would be reduced. *Yes, no. Yes, no.* I weighed the options. "He should participate in the clinical trial," I told the physician, who promptly made a telephone call that would determine if Dad would receive the experimental drug or not. Unfortunately, we were told that he did not meet all the criteria to be in the study.

I broke the news to Dad, who was cringing from pain, even though he was receiving morphine. Now what? Over 40 percent of first heart attacks are fatal. I didn't know that statistic then. Still, I had a sense there might only be minutes left, so I finally called my mother and broke the news. I didn't want to rob her of the chance to say good-bye. We decided not to wake up my younger brother John, a junior in high school sleeping at home, because he was scheduled to take the SATs that morning. Later, he too, would become a doctor, but for now he was my little brother and I needed to shield him. Then I went back to Dad's bedside and took his hand. "You're a great dad," I began to stammer. I could feel myself losing it. He turned to me from behind the veil of tubes. "Don't start to show it," he said.

I was taken aback, but I got it. The last thing Dad needed was for me to be a window to the end. He wanted me to be strong. But how could I be? To pull myself together, I took refuge in the nearest restroom. There, I was struck by the hospital-regulation basic white sink with overhanging mirror. Feeling a familiar tug from my Catholic upbringing, I couldn't help but notice how much the fixtures looked like an altar. Kneeling on the bathroom's chilly tile, I pleaded with God not to take my father. *Please don't let him die.* Hopefully, at a time when there was doubtless ample suffering in the world, I could garner God's attention. I didn't know what else to do.

I just couldn't imagine what I would do without my father. Dad had been my support for so much of my life, through all my forays into competitive sports, from grade school through medical school. And I still needed him. My mother was proud of me, and always there for me, but I someday wanted to walk down the aisle at my wedding on my father's arm.

Everybody deals with crises differently, and when my mother arrived at the hospital, my father got a scolding. "Joe, I told you not to smoke," she said. It was true. My father had acquired the habit during his army days, and we were all constantly hounding him to quit. And even though Dad was a mail carrier who got lots of exercise, his physical fitness didn't override his smoking. Interestingly, just prior to his heart attack, he was told his total cholesterol was normal. But we would later learn that he actually had low levels of HDL, the "good" cholesterol that protects the heart against heart disease, which wasn't reflected in Dad's "total" number. Admittedly, Dad's diet could have been better. Even walking several miles a day couldn't undo all those years of Italian sausage!

Wisdom 911

I learned so many important lessons on that early morning in May, right before I was to start my clinical training and the second two years of medical school: seeing a heart attack happening and experiencing such a huge loss of control, having to make dire life-or-death decisions in an instant; feeling I was about to lose someone I loved—without the chance to tidy up affairs or really tell him how much he meant to me. With heart disease, the leading killer of both men and women in the United States, it's no doubt that countless people experience a similarly frightening scenario, whether it be a stranger on the subway, a close family member or a coworker who was just a minute ago typing away at his desk. We all hear stories. And based on the statistics, there's a good chance that one day that person could be you or your father, mother, spouse, friend or grandparent—either as victim or rescuer.

What could Dad or we have done differently to avoid this medical crisis? As it turns out, plenty! Because, despite all of the scary statistics surrounding heart disease, there's a fact that most of us overlook: it is preventable. It doesn't have to happen to you or someone you love. If you play your cards right by knowing and taking a few small steps, which I'll discuss throughout this book, you can avoid being the one in the emergency room who is making those tough medical decisions or undergoing treatment. And that's my mission: to help you take action to prevent heart disease and live a long, healthy life.

Your Heart—The Inside Story

But first, a biology lesson. To defeat heart disease—public health enemy number one—you should get familiar with your heart. Your heart is the most important muscle in your body because if it stops working, so does everything else. Here's a brief job description of what your heart does and what can go wrong.

Each day, your heart works hard for you, continuously pumping blood throughout your body, whether you're reading quietly or racing for the bus. About the size of your fist, your heart beats (expands and contracts) an average of one hundred thousand times each day and circulates about two thousand gallons of blood. Because the heart is the epicenter of your body, it gets fed first with blood from coronary arteries. They're responsible for keeping the heart well supplied with a lifeline of oxygenated, nutrient-rich blood.

During a heart attack, the blood supply to the heart becomes severely reduced or cut off because one or more arteries become blocked by a blood clot. Blood clots don't happen by themselves. When arterial plaque is soft and filled with cholesterol, it builds up in arteries and becomes unstable and inflamed. Through a complex sequence of biochemical events, it then develops a crack or fissure, which releases substances that encourage clot formation. To be specific, it's usually a clot attached to a plaque that causes a heart attack because no blood can get through to supply oxygen and other nutrients to the working heart muscle. That's why risk factors for plaque buildup—inflammation and clotting—are important to be aware of and track.

When a heart attack occurs and blood flow is restricted, the heart muscle may not be able to effectively propel blood to the rest of the body, including the lungs. Subsequently, cells in the heart muscle don't receive enough life-giving oxygen and begin to die, which starts happening in just a few minutes. Because heart cells don't regenerate, the loss is permanent and can cause disability or even death. Time is of the essence. When symptoms of a heart attack occur, the clock starts ticking. In fact, half of the deaths from heart attacks occur in the first three or four hours after symptoms begin.

But if we take steps to recognize heart disease early on, it's much more treatable. It's akin to breast cancer and mammography screening. It's better to be aware of the signs and symptoms of heart disease and take heed by alerting your doctor as soon as possible that something's up. Awareness is key.

Know the Warning Signs

Over half of those who die suddenly from a heart attack—two-thirds of whom are women—have no previous recognized symptoms. Like my father, many people don't even know they have heart disease until the heart sets off its flare guns in the form of a heart attack. In the United States, heart disease will strike an estimated 1.2 million this year alone according to the National Heart, Lung, and Blood Institute, and kill over five hundred thousand. But, in retrospect, the signs may have been there but missed or dismissed. The symptoms, especially in women, can be sneaky.

Knowing these warning signs may someday save a life—and it may be yours or that of someone you love.

Common Signs and Symptoms of Heart Disease:

- **Chest discomfort or pain (angina).** This is the most typical symptom of heart disease. It's usually discomfort in the center of the chest or an uncomfortable pressure or pain that lasts for more than a few minutes or goes away and comes back. Other symptoms include heaviness, tightness, pain, burning, pressure or squeezing, usually behind the breast bone (sternum). These symptoms might radiate down the left arm or to the jaw or back.

- **Shortness of breath.** The feeling that you can't catch your breath is another classic sign of an impending heart attack. It often accompanies chest discomfort, but it can occur alone or before the chest pain starts.
- **Sweating (or diaphoresis).** Many patients, like my father, break out in a cold sweat; feeling clammy is a classic sign of a heart attack. It usually accompanies chest pain.

Medically known as a myocardial infarction, a heart attack is a medical emergency. We now realize that the best thing you can do if you or someone you know has chest pain is to immediately call 911 or your local emergency services (if 911 is not available in your area) because the time between the onset of symptoms and getting treatment is a critical determinant of survival. Don't wait. Far too many lives are lost because individuals are unsure of what's wrong, not realizing that time is critical. Clearly, it's better to be safe than sorry. Emergency services personnel can begin treatment as soon as they arrive.

When you call 911, you may be instructed to have the person experiencing symptoms chew one noncoated adult or two baby aspirin (if he or she is conscious), which helps improve the chances of survival by reducing the clot in the artery. If you're not instructed to use aspirin, do it anyway (as long as there's no aspirin allergy). But don't make the mistake of many and chew the aspirin, then wait for the pain to subside before making your 911 call. Pick up the phone first.

Also, check the time your symptoms began, so you can tell medical personnel. Why is timing so important? Remember the clot busters I mentioned in conjunction with my father's heart attack? Thanks to research, thrombolytic therapy and/or percutaneous coronary intervention (i.e. angioplasty) is now standard treatment for heart attack patients. Thrombolytics help preserve the heart muscle by dissolving clots that block an artery, which restores blood flow, like unkinking the garden hose. But here's the catch: for clot busters to be most effective, you need to receive them as soon as possible after the start of heart attack symptoms and preferably within one hour. Unfortunately, research shows the average patient with a heart attack waits two hours before seeking medical care after symptoms start. Don't take a "wait and see" approach because rapid action and intervention can not only save heart muscle, but possibly your life!

Less Common Warning Signs of Heart Disease

Heart attacks don't always give themselves away with classic signs. Sometimes symptoms are subtler. These less-common indicators of heart disease are considered atypical because most people experience more traditional signs. However, women are more likely to have atypical symptoms than are men. I've had many female patients recount how unusually tired they felt, for example, for about a month prior to their heart attacks. Tell your doctor if you have any of these symptoms:

- Unexplained fatigue
- Dizziness/light-headedness
- Headache
- Upset stomach/nausea
- Rapid heartbeat
- Feeling of impending doom

Some of these symptoms sound common. We all may have experienced them at one time or another. How do we know when to be concerned and seek medical care? First of all, note whether the symptoms occur with physical exertion or emotional strain. If the symptoms disappear with rest, they're more worrisome for heart disease. For example, I've had patients describe headaches that came on whenever they exerted themselves. That's an atypical symptom of heart disease that should be evaluated, especially if you have a family history or risk factors for heart disease.

Are the symptoms progressive in nature? If they're coming on more frequently or lasting longer, it may suggest unstable heart disease or a type of crescendo angina. I had a patient with frequent headaches that were increasing in severity. None of the physicians he saw could find anything wrong. Sure enough, he ended up having a heart attack and came to me after the fact to see how to prevent it from recurring. The first thing we talked about was recognizing that once you have an atypical symptom, that's most likely the way your heart disease is going to manifest itself again. That's Mother Nature's specific way of telling you that your heart isn't getting enough oxygen or blood. Anytime this patient has increasing headaches, he is on high alert to take it seriously and contact me.

Your Heart Disease Prevention "Coach"

As the director of Preventive Cardiology for NewYork-Presbyterian Hospital of Columbia and Cornell Universities in New York City, my life's work is to enhance the heart health of my patients and the public through high-quality and novel clinical service, research and educational programs. Inspired by my father's experience, I'm particularly committed to a family-centered approach to prevention. There's plenty of information out there about how to reduce your chances of having a heart attack, but sometimes your doctor may not talk to you about it. In medical school, we're trained to treat acute problems, with much less focus on how to prevent them. After I finished my internal medicine residency training, I pursued a fellowship in preventive cardiology so I could fill knowledge gaps in prevention that I knew someday might save a life, even of someone in my own family.

As a clinician, researcher and daughter, I've seen firsthand what happens when people take their health for granted. Professionally, I've witnessed the challenges well-intentioned patients have with incorporating positive lifestyle changes—and making them stick. I've also seen people die, or have their loved ones die, because of denial and lack of knowledge about how to prevent heart disease. It's devastating to lose someone we love too early in life, especially due to something preventable like heart disease. But why do we often wait until it's almost too late? That question took root on that May morning during my father's heart attack.

My passion for a career in preventive cardiology was further galvanized when, as an attending physician at the Syracuse Veterans Administration Hospital, I treated many veterans who had diseases and conditions—from diabetes and obesity to high cholesterol and high blood pressure—that resulted from poor lifestyle habits. I felt ill equipped to counsel these patients on the importance of eating better, getting more exercise and quitting smoking. The field of preventive cardiology was just emerging in the late 1980s when I was setting out; the medical profession was just beginning to make the connection between improving health habits and reducing disease risk. Even today, my own research shows doctors don't feel very effective in helping their patients reduce their risk of heart disease. That's why public awareness and education programs are so important. Knowing this, I sought a master's degree in public health and a Ph.D. in epidemiology. I realized that I needed more formal research training to find out the best ways to help doctors and patients alike.

Now, as the president of the American Society for Preventive Cardiology and the third woman in history to be chair of the American Heart Association Council on Epidemiology and Prevention, I'm so grateful to be in a position to forge a national research and public health agenda in prevention, and to develop strategies to translate science into real-life practice. I'm funded by the National Institutes of Health and have received early and mid-career research awards from the National Heart, Lung, and Blood Institute. I'm committed to seeing the tremendous advances in science used to improve public health.

Consider that an estimated 64 million Americans have one or more forms of cardiovascular disease (CVD), which includes acute heart attack, stroke and other forms of vascular disease throughout the body. While there are many forms of heart disease—from valve infections such as endocarditis to arterial conditions such as peripheral arterial disease—I'm going to focus on preventing atherosclerotic CVD, or hardening of the arteries, which is the main cause of heart attacks. The good news is that most of what we do to prevent heart attacks also helps prevent strokes and the hardening of other arteries throughout the body. According to the American Heart Association, heart disease kills more Americans than cancer, AIDS and drunk driving combined. I firmly believe that if we don't do more to personally combat CVD for ourselves and our families, it's going to prematurely claim the lives of millions more.

Our children are especially at risk for heart disease. Naturally, we want our kids to be healthy and stay that way throughout adulthood, but with tempting vending machines infiltrating schools and physical education programs being cut or eliminated across the country, it's no wonder that almost 9 million U.S. kids are now overweight or obese.

The problem doesn't end once the braces come off. Overweight kids have as much as an 80 percent chance of staying that way as adults and suffering from weight-related health problems earlier on, such as type 2 diabetes and, you guessed it, CVD. Given the staggering statistics and all that the medical profession knows about heart disease, we aren't doing enough to prevent the onslaught. Knowledge isn't enough. It's going to take a personal commitment. Let this book be your wake-up call to action.

In *Heart to Heart*, I'm going to have a personal discussion with you about CVD—not only as a researcher and clinician, but also as a daughter, wife and mother. I'll present a family-centered approach—and I use the term family liberally for whatever your circle of support and influence is. Like it or not, studies show that health habits emanate from the top down, and in this book, you're at the top. If you practice heart-healthy habits, so will your spouse, significant others, children, friends and anyone else you may touch. If you're taking care of your parents or other elders, they're apt to take your lead as well. It's a big responsibility, but some-body's gotta do it. But don't be afraid; I'll give you plenty of help for steering everyone in the right direction. (There's a reason why my sons, who are twelve and fifteen years old, selected a Mother's Day card that referred to me as "the advice channel.")

The chapters in *Heart to Heart* represent a distilled version of my twenty years of practice and ongoing education since medical school. I incorporate the ways I try to keep my own family healthy. In the following pages, I'll help you learn how to effectively:

- Make health—yours and that of your family—your top priority.
- Assess your CVD risk and genetic susceptibility, based on your personal and family medical history.
- Manage two major and common risk factors for CVD: high blood pressure and high cholesterol, and help your family do so as well.
- Understand the lifestyle risk factors that contribute to CVD, including obesity, smoking, stress, poor diet and lack of exercise, and how much of an impact making just small steps in the right direction can help.
- Motivate your loved ones to exercise regularly and eat a heart-healthy diet.

- Grasp the new heart-health guidelines and understand what they mean for you and your family.

- Get a big-picture perspective on heart health, including how seemingly unimportant habits, like routinely taking time for yourself, can actually help keep this major killer at bay.

- Talk to your doctor about the diagnostic tests you may need to improve your odds if your family or personal medical history is stacked against you, and other effective ways to help your doctor help you.

I'm also going to help you:

- Understand alternative/complementary therapies for CVD. From belladonna to yohimbine, herbal therapy is an area of treatment you may be investigating. I'll give you my take on this emerging field of medicine in relation to CVD prevention and discuss the potential efficacy and the risk of other over-the-counter therapies, such as antioxidants, multivitamins and other supplements.

- Learn about major blood pressure, cholesterol and diabetes drugs for when lifestyle isn't enough to minimize your CVD risk. I'll also provide a detailed discussion on CVD drugs you may have heard about, including statins, ACE inhibitors/ARBs, beta-blockers, aspirin therapy and other blood thinners/antiplatelet agents.

- Put prevention into action by role-modeling healthy lifestyle habits for your family.

Throughout, I'll share lessons learned over the years from my patients who became my teachers, and my own personal experiences as a physician-scientist, wife, mother and daughter, and how I try to practice what I teach. I'll share with you the life skills I've tried to arm my sons with that I hope someday they'll pass down, too, just like a cherished family recipe. You, too, may be the cog in the wheel of your family's heart health, and through a family-centered approach, I hope to help you keep moving in the right direction.

Boomers at Risk

Contrary to popular belief, although the risk of CVD increases with age, it's not *only* a disease of the old. In fact, baby boomers—those born between 1946 and 1964—are especially at risk, because that's when the disease tends to start—in middle age—although often silently, at first.

CVD doesn't discriminate based on income or celebrity status. We all know someone with CVD, even if we don't know them personally. Former president Bill Clinton, for example, who was just fifty-eight when he underwent successful quadruple coronary bypass surgery at our hospital in September 2004, is a heart disease survivor and boomer. President Clinton was fortunate because he got medical intervention before having a heart attack, which might have been fatal. It was a wake-up call for him and millions of Americans around his age. If it can happen to a former president who has access to the best medical care in the world, it can happen to any one of us. The good news is that just like the former president, we can adjust and make positive lifestyle changes that can save us.

If you're a baby boomer like Bill Clinton and me, you're one of seventy-six million Americans at an age in which CVD should be on your radar screen. It's a disease that threatens to kill a majority of our generation. In fact, 34 percent of men (5.6 million) and 29 percent of women (6.3 million) between the ages of forty-five and fifty-four already have CVD. According to the Centers for Disease Control and Prevention, that percentage increases to approximately half the U.S. population between the ages of fifty-five and sixty-four (12.1 million). Bottom line: if you're a boomer, you're not too young for CVD. In fact, now's the time to take steps to prevent the full-blown onset of it.

Wake Up Before It's Too Late

For me, it wasn't too late. In the end, my prayers were answered. Dad's heart wasn't extensively damaged by the heart attack in 1982. He survived that, as well as bypass surgeries of the heart, the legs and the carotid arteries feeding the brain. At seventy-six and married fifty years to my mom, he enjoys playing golf and being with his grandchildren. My two boys love to laugh at his jokes and get lessons on how to play pool—and above all, they think he is "really cool." I wish all stories had such a happy ending.

Unfortunately, many don't. I'll never forget the letter from a ten-year-old boy who donated $400 to the University of Michigan Division of Cardiology, where I served as director of Preventive Cardiology. The letter struck a chord because it echoed how I felt about my own father, and my older son happened to also be ten at the time. The boy was getting ready to go to school when the phone rang and his mother answered. When she put the phone down, she had to tell her son that his father had died of a heart attack during his business trip. He would never come home. To this day, reading his letter is difficult for me to get through. The fourth-grader wrote:

> . . . *so in this envelope is an amount of $400.00. I hope this money will help stop heart disiese* [sic] *and save someone's life. You don't relieze* [sic] *how much something means to you until it's gone. The time we had together I wouldn't sell for the world. I would give anything to have just one more day with him.*

Many patients, like this boy's father, don't get another shot. And that's the problem with heart disease. You don't always get a warning or the opportunity to put everything in order or the chance to prevent what didn't have to kill you in the first place. I have dedicated my career to heart disease prevention because I don't think any child should ever have to get that phone call. Here was a little boy, putting on his backpack, running out the door to school. He didn't get to grow up with his father or even say good-bye. This isn't how it has to happen. Knowledge is the power to change our lives as we know them. Action is the ability to change how we live. Congratulations for taking the first step to a long and healthy life.

THREE KEYS TO YOUR HEART

We'll complete this and every chapter with three key points I hope you'll remember about preventing heart disease. Three is a favorite number for me not just because I love triathlons, which I'll talk about more in the exercise chapter, but because I have a habit of summarizing the most important facts from any lecture I've heard or given down to three. Here are three from this chapter I hope you'll take to heart.

1. **Don't think it can't happen to you.** If heart disease affects over sixty-four million Americans, you or someone you love could easily be one of them. One American dies of cardiovascular disease every thirty-three seconds. The good news is that heart disease is preventable. You don't have to become a statistic.
2. **Know the symptoms.** The symptoms of heart attacks are: chest pain, shortness of breath, pain radiating down the arm or through the jaw, neck or back, or cold sweating. Be aware of these less common symptoms, too, which may signal a heart attack is on its way: unexplained fatigue, dizziness/light-headedness, nausea, headache, rapid heartbeat, a feeling of impending doom.
3. **Don't wait.** The greater the time delay between identifying symptoms and getting to an emergency room, where lifesaving drugs and interventions are available, the greater the chances a heart attack will lead to extensive heart damage. It's what we call "time to needle." Fast treatment can mean the difference between life and death. If you or someone you know is experiencing symptoms of a heart attack, call 911 or your local emergency services immediately. Often they can start life-saving treatment even before you get to the hospital, so it's important they transport you. Remember, when symptoms start, so does the clock.

Chapter

2

Partnering with Your Doctor for Prevention

"Like the body that is made up of limbs and organs, all mortal creatures are dependent upon one another."

—Hindu proverb

To prevent CVD, I think it's important to see your doctor once a year for a "well-adult" checkup. That's because we know that if we can catch something early, even before there are symptoms, there's a much greater likelihood that we can treat it and keep it from progressing. That goes for CVD as well as for cancer, diabetes and a host of other conditions that can sneak up on you, especially as you get older.

Every year around my birthday, I heed my own advice and give myself a present: a trip to the doctor—no matter what, even if I feel just fine and have all year—to check on the status of my own health. It's not a big deal, really. But getting everyone to do the same is one of the greatest challenges we face in the field of pre-vention. As patients and consumers, it seems that it's ingrained in us to go to the doctor only when we're sick, not when we're well (or seemingly so). But I've heard it all from my patients when they finally do come in to see me. Some are perfectly healthy and just want that confirmed. Others are experiencing subtle signs or won-der if what they're feeling is a symptom. They've been unexplain-ably tired lately or notice they now become short of breath even just going up stairs with a bag of groceries. Still, they've put off a visit because, as some have told me, "I didn't want to spend the money." Sometimes preventive care isn't covered by health insur-ance. Some say a preventive visit feels silly or neurotic. "I didn't want to seem like a hypochondriac," another patient said. And while it's true that there are those who are among the "worried well," or overly concerned about their health, they're by far the exception. Others tell me they hesitated to come in because they didn't want to waste my time, but finally, a concerned spouse, sib-ling or friend made the appointment for them and even came along. As I've noticed with many of my patients, accompanying reluctant loved ones to the doctor can be an effective way to finally get them through the office door. It's a way to be the "heart keeper" of your family.

If any of these scenarios sound familiar, believe me when I say a preventive care visit is worth it. It's an appropriate use of my time, and most physicians appreciate it when you're proactive. We applaud patients who embrace and take charge of their health. Even more important, a preventive care visit helps doctors and patients get to know each other so if there is a problem in the future, you have a physician to call, someone with whom you feel comfortable. A checkup means much more than lab work, a check of your blood pressure, a few deep breaths and a tap on the knee.

Need another nudge? Let's revisit the statistics. Over sixty-four million Americans have some form of CVD, but only one-third know it. Roughly fifty million Americans have high blood pressure, but because it has no symptoms, one-third aren't aware of their risk. Finally, one American dies of CVD every thirty-three seconds. Over half of those who die suddenly of CVD had no previous symptoms. But they might be alive today had they simply known CVD was a possibility. A preventive health checkup might have saved their lives.

Don't Go It Alone

Be the captain of your own ship. If you haven't seen a physician in over a year, or if you're experiencing occasional symptoms of CVD such as shortness of breath, discomfort or pain in your chest or one or both arms, neck, jaw or stomach, or anything else you consider unusual or different, especially upon exertion, make an appointment with your doctor today. In fact, I encourage you to write your appointment date and time in the space that follows.

My preventive health appointment is scheduled for:

_____   _____
Date   Time

Finding the Right Doctor

Of course, if you don't have a primary care physician or a gyne-cologist (the primary care physician for many women), the first step is to find a doctor you respect and are comfortable with. What

I suggest is asking your family and friends or other doctors for recommendations. Local hospitals, medical schools and medical
societies can usually provide the names of primary care physicians
and specialists. Then, find out more about those recommended by
checking their credentials with your health insurance plan. You
can also look them up in the *American Medical Directory &
Physicians Guide* at your local library or visit the American Medical
Association Web site at *www.ama-assn.org*. The doctors you choose
should be board certified, which means they have completed specific training in their fields and have passed required tests. If you
need a specialist, which may be the case if you've been diagnosed
with CVD, many major hospitals have referral services that can
help you identify an affiliated physician with the expertise you
need. Disease-specific Internet message boards, chat rooms and e-
mail listserv discussions can also be a good way to get the names,
telephone numbers and e-mail addresses of top medical specialists from across the country. Take this search seriously. Personally,
I think we should spend at least as much time finding the right
doctor as we do the perfect outfit for a special occasion, which
may have only a one-time use. Shouldn't the person who is going
to be guiding us toward optimal health be someone we've actually
investigated? It's worth the legwork when you find a doctor you're
compatible with, someone who is willing to talk with you and listen. Consider interviewing several doctors. I have patients come to
me all the time who have recently "fired" their doctors because
they wanted to find someone who would spend more time with
them, listen well and focus on prevention.

Doctor Shopping

When choosing a doctor, I think it's important to choose a primary care physician or specialist who emphasizes health as much as disease. There are plenty of wonderful doctors who are paying attention to lifestyle risk factors and the latest preventive guidelines and who are good role models. It's also well documented that some aren't, so you should shop around. When interviewing a doctor, you might say, "I'm concerned about heart disease. How important do you think prevention is for treating CVD risk factors, like high blood pressure and high blood cholesterol?" Then compare the responses you get. If the doctor is aware of the latest CVD prevention guidelines, you're on the right track.

Helping Your Doctor Help You

As a physician whose practice is dedicated to CVD prevention, I often see patients who are dissatisfied with their cardiologist or their primary care physician because they're not getting the time they want or a feeling of support. That's a valid complaint, but I have to say that in today's medical climate, time *is* an issue with the medical profession as a whole. A typical doctor's office visit may last just ten minutes. That's ten minutes to talk with your doctor about why you're there, undergo a physical exam, get a diagnosis (if relevant), and develop a treatment or prevention plan. It certainly doesn't sound like enough time to get it all done, but it can be if you're prepared and organized.

To help you get the most of your ten minutes with your doctor
—and *psst*—garner even more time with your doctor if you need it
(it's possible), here's what I suggest:

Be on time. Although the medical profession has a reputation
for keeping patients waiting, many physicians are on time for
appointments. If I'm on time and you're not, what tends to happen is that your appointment gets pushed down the line. You then
run the risk being rushed.

Bring your records. It saves a lot of time when you bring in relevant past records and the results of any recent lab tests or diagnostic studies. This prevents the doctor from leaving the room to
track down the information or find a staff member to help. It's
much less disruptive to the visit if you bring your records or send
them in advance.

State the facts, and let the doctor diagnose. At the start of your
visit, often the nurse or doctor will ask, "What's your chief complaint?" because that's how we're taught to start an evaluation in
medical school. We often have to document the chief complaint
for billing and reimbursement purposes as well. Be clear and as
specific as you can about your symptoms, if you have any, and
when they started. Don't hold back. Something you think is
minor—a twinge here or there—could affect your treatment or
prevention plan. Conversely, something you think is serious might
be easily remedied. Also, when your doctor walks in and asks why
you're there, it's best not to state a guess, such as, "I think I have
heart disease." It would be better to say, for example, "I'm concerned about my risk for heart disease because my uncle just had
a heart attack. I want to be checked out." Then be prepared to discuss any symptoms you might have, your medical history and your
lifestyle.

The chief-complaint framework doesn't really work for preventive health visits because you might not have any complaints, let

alone a major one. That's okay. When you're asked why you're there, just say, "I'm here for a preventive health checkup." If you've been experiencing any symptoms, though, mention how severe they are, if the pattern has been changing, and if they're brought on by exertion or stress. For example, you might say, "I'm here because I have a shooting pain in my right arm that started a week ago. Sometimes it's so painful, I have to stop what I'm doing."

It's a good idea to bring along a notebook containing your medical and family health history, which I'll discuss in more detail in chapter 3. This is especially helpful on a first-time visit, when most physicians do a personal and family health history intake.

Your notebook should include dates and reasons for previous doctor visits, test results, immunizations, childhood illnesses, past medications you've taken and those you're now taking, and their doses and any reactions they may have caused. In addition, you should list any chronic conditions you have (diabetes, arthritis, etc.) and the current health status or cause of death of your parents and grandparents. If you've spent time in the hospital, include a copy of your discharge lab work summary. Also bring records of tests or surgeries. Medical office staff can help you obtain copies of these documents.

Speak up. The goal of the visit to the doctor is to get your questions, issues and condition (if relevant) out in the open. Even if a subject or question is embarrassing, if it's pertinent to the reason for your doctor's visit, mention it. The information you provide about your condition or lifestyle could be a key element to your treatment. Some of my patients diagnosed with heart disease, for example, have asked me if having sex will cause a recurrent heart attack. That can be a tough question to ask for some. (Answer: It's usually perfectly fine to have sex even if you have established heart disease.) Also, be honest about whether you will follow or are following your doctor's recommendations—or those from anyone on your health care team, which may include a registered dietitian (R.D.). If something's not working, we want to know so we can brainstorm more realistic solutions to help you stay on track. Keep in mind that you're not a failure if you haven't followed doctor's orders in the past. There are many reasons why many patients don't, and sometimes it's because the doctor didn't make it clear how important it was to follow his/her advice. Remember, we're here to help you achieve optimal health. We're not here to judge you.

Bring your meds. If you take any medications, including anything over-the-counter, bring them with you. This can help your doctor avoid prescribing something that may adversely interact with what you already take. The doctor may also recommend discontinuing unproven therapies, even if they seem "natural" and harmless.

Summarize your visit. As your visit comes to a close, it's important to review the answers to any questions you brought with you. You should have a clearer picture of your diagnosis, prognosis and treatment plan before you walk out the door. If you don't, ask your doctor to go over it with you.

Exam Time

To avoid breaking your doctor's concentration, let your doctor work in silence while performing your physical exam. When the exam is over, it's time to ask, "Does everything look normal?" or, "How am I doing?" More specific questions are even better. If you're in for a preventive health checkup, you'll likely be sent off to the lab for blood work to check your cholesterol profile and other "numbers."

Wrap up your visit by asking what the next steps are likely to be. In some cases, it may be having blood work done, then getting a

A NOTE FROM DR. LORI:
SIZING UP YOUR SYMPTOMS

Your doctor may be trained in medicine, but you know your body better than anyone. To gain clarity before your doctor's visit, make a detailed list of specific questions to ask the doctor, putting the main symptoms or concerns at the top. Bring the list with you so you won't forget anything. Include on it the following information:

- If you have any pain or possible symptoms of heart disease, when they started and how often they occur.
- Whether the pattern of symptoms has been changing or worsening.
- Whether the symptoms are related to stress or a specific action, such as only when you run for the bus or lift something heavy.
- How the symptoms interfere with your daily life. For example, do they keep you from going to work, or are they keeping you awake at night?
- If it's a preventive visit, and you don't have symptoms, be prepared to discuss your family and personal medical history as well as your lifestyle.

call from a nurse or the doctor stating your results. When you get the call, don't settle for generalities, such as, "Your cholesterol is fine." Get specifics so you can know your numbers. Keep in mind that in addition to your body mass index (BMI) and waist circumference, you want to know your total cholesterol, LDL cholesterol, HDL cholesterol, triglycerides, blood pressure and fasting blood glucose. That said, you may need to ask, "What is my HDL ("good") level, my LDL ("bad") level and my total cholesterol level? What is my triglyceride level?" and so on. I'll discuss each of these risk factors in chapter 3. Remember, knowledge is power—and the first step toward preventing CVD.

Now it's time to discuss a treatment or prevention plan with your doctor, which may involve a follow-up phone call or visit. When discussing your next steps, ask what symptoms you'll likely experience if the situation worsens and what else you can do to improve treatment or reduce your risk factors, such as changing your diet or exercise regimen. Be sure to consider asking the following:

- Am I at high, intermediate or low risk for CVD?
- Is there anything in my family history that increases my risk of heart disease?
- What should my cholesterol levels be, and how can I improve them?
- What should my blood pressure be, and how can I improve it?
- Do I have diabetes, or am I at risk of developing diabetes?
- How much physical activity should I get?
- Do I need to get a stress test before I start exercising?
- What type of diet is appropriate for me?
- Should I take aspirin to prevent a heart attack?
- How often should I have my risk factors checked?

Finally, if you're given a prescription, ask what the medication does and what side effects you may experience. Also, establish a time frame for following up, and inquire whether the follow-up should be done by phone or in person. You'll also want to ask if your health plan covers the recommended treatment (if applicable). And remember, saying "Thanks for your help" at the conclusion of your visit helps build good rapport, which is in your best interest.

So Many Questions, So Little Time

To help you take charge of your health, here are other questions, recommended by the American Heart Association, you might pose on your first and subsequent visits to the doctor, based on your risk factors.

High Blood Pressure

- What is my blood pressure, and how can I reach or maintain a healthy level?
- How often should I have my blood pressure checked?
- Should I be on blood pressure–lowering medicine in addition to following a more healthful lifestyle?

Obesity

- How can I reach or maintain a healthful weight?
- What kind of physical activity should I do?

Smoking

- How does smoking affect my heart health?
- How can I quit smoking?
- How can I avoid possible weight gain after I quit smoking?

Diabetes

- What is diabetes, and how might it affect my heart health?
- What are the risk factors for diabetes?
- Diabetes runs in my family. How can I prevent it?
- I have diabetes. How can I control it?
- I have diabetes, and I know that increases my risk of heart disease and stroke. Should I be on a statin and/or an ACE inhibitor?

What Questions Will You Ask Your Doctor?

Go ahead. Write them here:

_____

_____

_____

_____

_____

A NOTE FROM DR. LORI:
GETTING MORE FACE TIME

Keep in mind that if you need more than ten minutes at your visit to ask your doctor questions, he or she will probably accommodate you if you ask questions in a non-threatening way, such as, "I know you're very busy, but I'm really trying to improve my cholesterol numbers, and I was wondering if you could be more specific about what they mean. Could you please help me?" Who could say no to that?

Housekeeping Notes: Getting It Write

A visit to your doctor can be stressful, which can impair your ability to listen and think clearly. Consequently, there's often a significant discrepancy between what you're told and what you hear. That's why it's a good idea to jot down the details about your condition and the prevention plan that your doctor mentions during the postexamination discussion, or the few minutes you spend talking with your doctor before leaving.

If your condition is particularly complex, bring your spouse or a family member or a friend along to help get the facts for you.

Having as much information as possible can help you ask questions on subsequent visits so you can make the most educated decisions regarding your health care and prevention plan. If you're not getting all the answers you want or need, or if the information is not presented in the way you can understand, don't be embarrassed to slow down the pace of the conversation and ask for an explanation.

Try not to leave the doctor's office without knowing what to do next. And don't forget to get the following instructions:

• How long you should take any prescribed or over-the-counter medication.

• Whether there are any foods, beverages or supplements you should avoid that might interfere with the effectiveness of your medications. (If applicable)

• How long it will be before you should start to feel better (if applicable).

• When to call your doctor if you don't feel better as expected (if applicable).

• When to schedule a follow-up appointment or blood work.

It's generally acceptable to call (or in some cases e-mail) your doctor or his/her assistant when you get home if you don't understand a medical concept or have a question that didn't occur to you at the time of the visit. But because doctors have only so much time to spend on the phone, try to avoid calling about an issue that's unrelated to your initial visit. If a new problem plagues you, it's better to make another appointment. Most of us don't like to treat patients over the phone unless it is a straightforward issue. This doesn't mean you should not call to find out if you should be seen and how quickly—that is perfectly okay.

Do Your Homework

Although it might sound like a lot of effort, researching your medical condition can enable you to discuss the matter with your doctor in more detail. You can also educate yourself about issues related to your condition that your doctor may not have time to discuss. To better understand your diagnosis, the Internet can be a useful tool but keep in mind the information obtained online is not always accurate. If you run across an important new study related to your condition, you might want to present it to your doctor. To save time, make a copy so your doctor can read the full text. Or send it to him or her in the mail. In fact, I love it when patients come to me with articles about their conditions they've looked up online and in the newspapers, with a list of detailed questions. That shows me they really care and want to make positive changes.

But keep in mind that the information you find online and elsewhere isn't the same as experience and education, which allows your doctor to put the information in context. In my experience, patients can go awry when they take the information they've gathered from the Internet or the latest report on the evening news as gospel. They want to know why I haven't prescribed a certain drug, test or treatment, even though the write-up in the newspaper about a particular new study says that's the thing to do.

What they may not realize is there are many individual circumstances that determine whether or not a particular test, treatment or drug is right for them. Moreover, the information they collect may not be relevant to them. The published results of a major clinical trial, for example, may seem significant, but if the population studied in the trial is different from you—if it's all men, say, and you're a woman—the effect of the intervention may not be so predictable in you. Taking a more active role in your health care can give you a feeling of control. But while you do that, remember that your doctor is still needed to filter and interpret new information based on the totality of evidence that's available to make clinical decisions. Medicine is a moving target. But it's rare that a single new study or report changes the way we practice. We have to place new data in the context of what we already know, and what we still don't know, to make informed recommendations. In the end, when the final decision to accept a treatment is made, the buck stops with you. But it's your doctor's professional judgment you're relying on. That's why it's important to select a credentialed physician whom you trust and have confidence in.

A NOTE FROM DR. LORI: GETTING YOUR DOCTOR'S TAKE ON THE LATEST STUDY

If you approach your doctor with information about your condition from the news or the newspaper, be prepared for the possible reality that he or she may not yet have heard about it. That's because patients often get some information before we do. We usually don't get a full research paper or the medical journal that discusses the latest "this just in" findings until a few days or so after the study results have been highlighted on the evening news. There's always a lag time. With that in mind, it's fine to alert your doctor to the latest news health alert, but he or she will need time to digest the material, place it into context of everything else that's out there, and consider the limitations of the study, which many consumers and medical reporters are not trained to do, so try to be patient.

Plan for Success

One of the winningest basketball coaches of all time, John Wooden, use to tell his players, "Failing to prepare is preparing to fail." I could not agree more. You must prepare for success in health as in life.

Health care is a team activity that involves you, doctors, nurses and other caregivers from family to neighbors. Your relationship with your doctor, especially, should be one in which you feel involved and take personal accountability for your own well-being. You shouldn't feel like you're simply following "doctor's orders." That's a paradigm that simply doesn't work anymore, especially with CVD prevention, which almost always involves lifestyle modification—in other words, *active* participation on your part. It pays to know the hows and whys, ask questions and get answers.

If you feel like a bystander in managing your condition and/or risk factors or feel intimidated, consider finding a different doctor. More patients are now seeking out doctors who are willing to listen to them and involve them in the process (they're out there!). All told, when dealing with your doctor, make this your motto for your CVD treatment and prevention plan: *Nothing about me without me.* That's an empowering message that helps keep you involved in the proactive process of maintaining a healthy heart because, ultimately, reducing your risk of CVD to live a stronger, healthier life requires a team-player mind-set on both your and your doctor's part.

Other Partners in Prevention

Because CVD prevention happens as much or more outside the doctor's office as it does within, it's helpful to engage other partners (in addition to your doctor) who can support you in your quest for optimal health. At New York–Presbyterian Hospital where I direct preventive cardiology, we developed a partner-in-prevention contract to help our patients achieve their goals. A partner in prevention is someone (family member/friend) who will support your efforts of living heart smart. I encourage you to take the time now to fill out your contract and team up with a prevention partner.

Photocopy this contract and distribute it to your loved ones so they can officially get with the program, too. Many of my patients who spend a lot of time working at their computers tell me they like to post theirs in a spot next to their computer screens, so they'll be sure to see it every day. Others have said that it has a special place right inside the cover of their daily planners. Where will you display yours?

When Second Opinions Are Good Medicine

If you've been diagnosed with CVD and/or you're facing major surgery or another major medical procedure, such as angioplasty and cardiac stenting, good news: for most major diseases, there are more treatment options than ever. But each treatment choice brings advantages and disadvantages and its own set of complications and possible side effects. That's why you might want to get a second medical opinion if you have a serious medical illness such as CVD. Without one, it can be more difficult to compare the different kinds of treatment available to you and make an informed, deliberate decision about your care. Studies show that for some diseases, as many as 50 percent of patients who go for a second opinion are offered a different treatment option than originally planned. Getting a second medical opinion can also be useful to confirm or change a diagnosis.

A second medical opinion is nothing more than seeing a different doctor who will review your medical history, including all diagnostic test results up to that point, perform a focused examination and talk with you about various treatment options available. You may be asked to undergo more or different medical tests—or not. Consider it another way to educate yourself about CVD. Getting a second opinion will improve your understanding of your treatment options and may even reinforce your confidence in your primary care physician if your initial diagnosis is confirmed. In any event, you'll get a slightly different perspective, which can be extremely useful in understanding your illness and taking responsibility for your own health care.

It isn't always necessary. You might not need a second opinion if you and your team of health care providers have explored all the treatment options, you have a clear understanding of the alternatives, and you've chosen a course of treatment everyone has agreed on and is comfortable with. In addition, if your situation is a medical emergency, it may not be wise to delay treatment for a second opinion.

On the other hand, if you feel you haven't received adequate information, or you've done research and think other options are available that haven't been offered, a second opinion is extremely important. But how should you go about getting a second opinion?

PERSONAL CONTRACT FOR HEART-SMART LIVING

I will make an effort to live heart smart by taking a small step toward achieving my prevention goals.

I will choose a specific behavior _____

to work on that will improve my heart health by _____.

My optimal goal is to _____.

I will succeed in meeting this goal by doing the following things:

_____

_____

_____

_____

I will achieve my optimal goal by ____ / ____ / ____.

When I meet my optimal goal, I will give myself a reward that is positive and makes me feel good.

When I _____, my reward will be

_____

_____

Your Signature   Date

_____

Signature of Your Partner in Prevention   Date

Team Up with Your Primary Care Physician

Getting a second opinion can be politically treacherous. Some patients, for example, worry about offending their primary care physicians, who are often the doctors making the initial diagnoses, and so try to get a second opinion without their knowledge. That's usually not the best route to take. Unless your primary care doctor is resistant to the idea, involve your doctor in the process. Your doctor should have full knowledge of what's going on in terms of your medical care and can often help make the arrangements for getting a second opinion. Don't worry about offending your doctor. Most primary care physicians aren't threatened by a second opinion if it's done in the spirit of being fully informed about a diagnosis and disease. In fact, they may be pleased to have patients get second opinions because, often, a second opinion reinforces a patient's confidence in the initial diagnosis and treatment plan.

To get an unbiased second opinion, it may be best to visit a different medical institution or medical group. For starters, get the names of specialists in several different medical groups from your doctor. Or approach your doctor with recommendations you've acquired on your own by networking with friends and relatives or from the Internet and other sources. You might say to your doctor, "My research has shown that this may be somebody who would be able to give me a second opinion, so I can make the best decisions for my health."

After you've made an appointment with the second physician, be prepared to do some legwork. Your medical records will probably be sent from your first physician to the second one, but you may be asked to gather your own X-rays and other diagnostic test results. There is such a thing as a "blind" diagnosis, in which you don't provide the secondary physician with your medical records, test results or diagnosis to avoid influencing the second opinion with previous information. That's not usually the best idea. I think all of your medical records and X-rays should be provided to the physician making the second medical opinion so the doctor has all information to make a fully informed decision about the treatment options at his/her fingertips.

There are second-opinion doctors who are comfortable making a long-distance diagnosis with just your medical records and lab tests. This may be convenient, especially if your second-opinion physician practices out of state. Still, try to meet with the doctor in person. In many ways, your options for health care are personal and individual. Some of your treatment options may depend on what a physician finds on a physical exam. Some may depend on how you feel about those options, your personal beliefs and circumstances, and the questions you ask. In general, I think it's important to meet with the physician face-to-face, if possible.

Insurance Coverage

Although coverage for health care varies nationally, most insurers pay for second opinions, especially if it comes from an in-network physician. In some states, second opinions are mandated. Check with your health plan regarding its second-opinion policies and the guidelines you need to follow. But if you're not covered for second medical opinions, don't let that necessarily stop you from getting one.

When a Second Opinion Differs

In many cases, a second opinion doesn't alter a diagnosis or treatment plan considerably. Still, the second opinion you receive could vary widely from the first. What to do? Go back to your physician and discuss how widely both opinions vary. Your doctor may be able to help you sort out your options and decide whether you need a third opinion. When diagnosed with a life-altering illness, you owe it to yourself and your loved ones to explore all of your options.

Three Keys to Your Heart

Here are three key points I hope you'll take to heart from this chapter:

1. **See your doctor even when you are well.** A yearly visit is one of the best ways to monitor your risk factors and your health status to ensure that CVD as well as other preventable conditions don't get a foothold. It's also helpful for building a relationship with your doctor, so you feel you have someone to turn to should something go wrong.
2. **Do your research.** Find a credentialed physician as your primary care provider whom you trust and feel comfortable with asking questions. If the chemistry isn't there, or you don't feel you're receiving the time or support you need, keep looking for someone who is a better fit. When it comes to preventing CVD, you should feel that you and your doctor have a shared mission.
3. **Be a proactive patient.** Prepare for your doctor visits by bringing a list of questions and giving your doctor the information he or she needs to make an accurate assessment of your health, such as an overview of your personal and family medical history and any symptoms you may be experiencing. Don't be afraid to question your doctor about your treatment or prevention plan or to present medical findings you come across that might be relevant to your situation. Remember, preventing CVD is a team effort.

Chapter

3

What's in a Number?

"Prediction is very difficult, especially about the future."

—Niels Bohr

Every so often, I encounter patients with no identifiable risk factors for heart disease, yet they have CVD. Why them? Caroline, an actress in her late fifties, fell into that category. I met her after she had triple bypass surgery. Caroline's doctor asked me to consult on her case to determine what might have caused her condition. "Where did I go wrong?" she asked me from her hospital bed. It was a good question. Caroline knew of no heart disease in her family. She seemed perfectly healthy—until she was rushed to the emergency room sweating, short of breath, with chest pain, signaling what later turned out to be arteries that were 90 percent blocked. "My cholesterol was fine," she insisted. She wanted answers, and so did her doctor, so she could go forward and not be blindsided by catastrophe again.

Pouring through her records, I saw that Caroline's gynecologist had noted a few years back that her HDL (the "good") cholesterol was okay. But according to the blood tests I performed, Caroline's HDL cholesterol was 42, which wouldn't have been so bad if she were a man. For men, an HDL cholesterol less than 40 (mg/dL) is considered a risk factor. But for women, HDL cholesterol less than 50 is considered suboptimal, and that was Caroline's problem. Due to her low HDL cholesterol, she had an increased risk of CVD that went undiagnosed for maybe ten to twenty years. "I wish I would have known I was actually in harm's way," she said to me. "I would have done anything to avoid needing bypass surgery."

I wish she had been properly informed, too, because once you are diagnosed with CVD, you are seven times more likely to have a heart attack or die of heart disease. Hopefully Caroline won't become that statistic. But now that she's aware of her risk factor—low HDL cholesterol—she can target it. Knowing your risk factors is so important for taking responsibility for your own health future—and to help your loved ones do the same. Remember, CVD is preventable if you have the foresight to fend it off before symptoms develop.

Know the Difference Between Good and Bad

As you may know, there are "good" and "bad" kinds of cholesterol, HDL and LDL. HDL is commonly called the "good" cholesterol because it tends to carry cholesterol away from the arteries and back to the liver, where it's passed from the body. HDLs remove excess cholesterol from plaque in arteries, thus slowing the buildup. On the other hand, too much of the "bad" LDL cholesterol in the blood, which the liver produces, can cause a buildup of plaque—cholesterol and fat—inside walls of the arteries. To tell the good stuff from the bad, just remember:

LDL = L is for Lousy; we want it Lower.
HDL = H is for Healthy; we want it Higher.

What Are <u>Your</u> Risk Factors?

The historian Francis Newton said, "I can stand what I know. It's what I don't know that frightens me." And when it comes to risk factors for CVD what you don't know can hurt you. It's not enough to know what the major risk factors for heart disease are. Each one of us should know our specific number and our risk. This is the most important first step in taking action to reduce risk. Low HDL cholesterol like Caroline's is just one of many risk factors for CVD. In fact, there are at least four hundred all told for heart disease, many of them genetic. Don't worry, I'm not going to cover all four hundred here because only a handful of risk factors are considered major and have proven therapies to reduce your risk. They're the ones I'll home in on in this chapter.

The following are nonmodifiable factors that increase your CVD risk. You can't do anything about them, but it's still good to be aware of them. If you know you're at increased risk, you can be extra vigilant with your lifestyle and other CVD risk factors that you can modify.

Age

The risk of heart attack and stroke increases with age. For women, heart disease is less common before age fifty-five than among older age groups. For men, like my father who was fifty-three when he had his heart attack, the disease becomes more common after age forty-five. Why does age up the odds for CVD? As we get older, so do our arteries. They become less pliable and less able to accommodate blood flow. The inner lining of the blood vessels, called the endothelium, can become damaged due to exposure to toxins (e.g., nicotine) in the blood, high cholesterol and high blood pressure. This early damage is called endothelial dysfunction, and it is important because it's one of the earliest signs that trouble is brewing. I like to think of endothelium as our "inner skin," and just as our outward appearance can reflect signs of aging, so does our "inner skin." In fact, it's been said, "You're only as old as your endothelium." Also, years of poor diet can lead to arteries becoming filled with cholesterol and plaque. Blood pressure tends to rise, as do cholesterol levels as the years go on. Until somebody finds a way to turn back the clock, we're all at heightened risk as the years round the bend.

Still, the process of heart disease—atherosclerosis, the condition in which plaque (thick, hard cholesterol [fatty] deposits) forms in artery walls to constrict or block blood flow, causing chest pain or even a heart attack—actually starts early. A landmark study in the *New England Journal of Medicine* in 1998, which involved the autopsies of 204 young people from two to thirty-nine years of age who had died from non-cardiac-related causes, showed that every one had fatty streaks and fibrous-plaque lesions, the precursers to plaque, so it is clear the seeds for CVD are planted early. That's why it's important to protect yourself and your loved ones from heart disease—the sooner the better.

Gender

Men are at risk for CVD about ten years earlier than women. Many of my male patients, for example, are in their late forties when they first come to see me; the majority of my female patients are nearing sixty, after they have had menopause.

Many scientists believe that the loss of estrogen at the time of menopause is what begins to increase the risk of CVD in women. Although loss of the possible protective effects of estrogen is an attractive hypothesis to explain the gender gap in CVD, hormone replacement therapy has not been shown to lower risk, so it's still a conundrum. Postmenopausal women have roughly the same risk of cardiac death as men who are ten years younger, unless they have diabetes. Having diabetes obliterates the female advantage for CVD.

Over the years, I have had many women patients in their forties with heart disease, and most of them have also had diabetes. Mandy was an overweight scientist in her forties who had diabetes and, after two failed angioplasties in the 1990s, needed bypass surgery. It is often the case that my sickest patients with CVD are relatively young women with diabetes.

Diabetes

Men and women with diabetes have an increased risk of CVD, and women more so than men. This gender difference may be attributable to the more damaging effects of high blood pressure and cholesterol (common problems associated with diabetes) on the blood vessels of women.

Obesity and physical inactivity are also associated with an increased risk of diabetes and CVD. Both lack of physical exercise and excess weight can make the body's insulin receptors less sensitive to the action of insulin—creating a state analogous to diabetes.

Race/Ethnicity

Mexican Americans are at an elevated risk of obesity-related diabetes, which may contribute to an increased risk of CVD. African Americans have moderate high blood pressure twice as often as Caucasians and severe high blood pressure three times as often. As a result, their risk for heart disease is greater. A striking example of the impact of race on health risk is that African American women, who have a 70 percent higher death rate due to heart disease than that of Caucasian women.

Heredity

Heart disease tends to run in families. If you have a first-degree male relative (father or brother) with heart disease before age fifty-five, as I do, or a first-degree female relative (mother or sister) with CVD before age sixty-five, you have a greater risk of developing heart disease yourself. It's a major red flag. However, having a blood relative with CVD at *any* age also heightens your risk of heart attack, although not as much as when it's a first-degree relative who was diagnosed with CVD prematurely. So just be aware, and take your health history seriously.

It's not just "bad" genes lurking in your family tree that should be a concern. Lifestyle plays a significant role in whether those genes get the chance to express themselves. Plus, risk-factor control can substantially reduce your risk, so your genes don't necessarily determine your destiny.

Other Conditions

You're also at increased risk for a future heart attack if you have a past history of heart disease or other arterial conditions, including peripheral arterial disease, chronic kidney disease, abdominal aortic aneurysm or cerebrovascular/carotid artery disease. A prior stroke also increases the risk of heart attack.

Take Advantage of Motivational Moments

Having a friend or relative hospitalized with CVD may be a "motivational moment," a period when we feel especially susceptible to CVD ourselves and are more likely to take preventive action. For example, when my Dad had his heart attack, that would have been a good time for my entire immediate family to get checkups to determine the status of our own heart health. Turns out my older brother also had a low HDL cholesterol just like my dad but he didn't find out about it until many years later, potentially losing precious time.

To harness these can-it-happen-to-me opportunities, at NewYork-Presbyterian Hospital Preventive Cardiology Program we started a free risk-factor screening and education program for family members and friends of patients hospitalized with CVD. The program, called PASSPORT to Heart Health for Families, is designed to help friends and family of those afflicted determine their own CVD risk and how to lower it at this teachable time. Of the initial 1,500 friends and family we screened, nearly 40 percent had more than three major risk factors for CVD. Fortunately, now they know and can do something about it.

But there's no need to wait until someone you know is diagnosed with CVD. Give yourself a birthday present every year, and go visit your doctor for a preventive exam. It's important to see your doctor regularly, not only to learn the status of your health but to establish a good relationship so that if something does happen to you, you'll feel comfortable calling to discuss it.

Nine Ways to Head Off Heart Attack

Okay, you're aware of the risk factors age, gender, race/ethnicity, heredity and prior diagnosis of CVD or diabetes. Now let's focus on the CVD risk factors you *can* control. I urge all of my patients to make these the mainstay of their prevention plan. By doing so, you can directly lower your risk of CVD, even, as I said, if you have a family history of the condition. National guidelines have been established to help those without cardiovascular disease prevent it from occurring. The following checklist is based on those recommendations. Use the checklist to mark off where you're doing well, and take note of what you need to work on.

❏ 1. Eat a Heart-Healthy Diet

To reduce your risk of CVD, your diet is a major player because we eat so often—at least three times a day—we have lots of opportunities to make the right food choices that can help our hearts stay strong and our arteries clear. We'll discuss diet in detail in chapter 6.

❏ 2. Exercise Every Day

To reduce your risk of CVD, do a minimum of thirty minutes of moderate-intensity aerobic exercise (such as brisk walking) on most, preferably all, days of the week. Recent guidelines suggest we all engage in sixty minutes of exercise daily to prevent weight gain. Like eating and drinking, exercise isn't optional. I consider it as vital as food and water—and shoe shopping. (Okay, I'm kidding, but you get the idea.) I'll discuss exercise in more detail in chapter 5.

Need motivation? Join Choose to Move, the free online twelve-week physical activity program sponsored by the American Heart Association at *www.americanheart.org*. Choose to Move covers practical ways to increase your physical activity and reduce your risk of CVD.

❏ 3. Keep Your Waist Whittled

To reduce your risk of CVD, keep tabs on your weight and your waistline. To be in a healthy range, your body mass index (BMI), which is a ratio of your weight in relation to your height, should be 18.5 to 24.9. To compute your BMI, log on to *http://nhlbisupport.com/bmi/bmicalc.htm*, and input your height and weight into the calculator. Record your BMI on the "Risk Factor Tracker" on page 62. It's also important to maintain a waist circumference of less than thirty-five inches (women) or less than forty inches (men). Body fat, especially in the midsection, increases the risk of CVD because it raises cholesterol and triglyceride levels as well as blood pressure and can increase your risk of diabetes. If you need to lose a few pounds, make a concerted effort to do so. Even losing just 10 percent of your total weight—that's twenty pounds if you weigh two hundred—can have a substantial effect on your overall risk of heart disease, which can translate to improved chances of survival.

❏ 4. Quit Smoking

If you smoke, stop completely. Each year, of the nearly one million American adults who die of CVD, one in five deaths are attributable to smoking. Cigarette and cigar smoke is toxic, containing carbon monoxide and other toxins that can cause CVD. When you stop smoking, your risk of heart disease caused by smoking is reduced by half—after only one year. After fifteen years of not taking a puff, your risk is similar to those who've never smoked. Need more motivation? Think of how much money you'll save by not buying cigarettes if you quit.

Steer clear of environmental tobacco smoke. Avoid bars and restaurants, for example, where smoking is still allowed. Sitting in the nonsmoking section doesn't work because smoke is insidious. "That's like trying to stay in the nonchlorinated section of the pool," I tell my patients. In other words, if smoke is allowed in a restaurant, the entire restaurant, even the nonsmoking section, is a smoking section.

Encourage your spouse and other family members to quit, and don't let anyone smoke in your house or in your car. I never let anyone smoke in mine; I don't even own any ashtrays. In the long run, secondhand smoke exposure may also increase your risk of heart disease and cancer, as well as your child's as an adult. Cigarette smoke has over four thousand toxins, most of which can irritate or kill cells in the body, depending on how much secondhand smoke you are exposed to, according to the Centers for Disease Control and Prevention's Office on Smoking and Health. Compared to adults, kids have an increased susceptibility to the harmful effects of secondhand smoke because they breathe at a faster rate; a child's natural detoxification system is also less developed.

Even if you and others avoid smoking around your kids, chemicals from cigarettes tend to hang in the air. They can imbed in your clothing, car seats, furniture and curtains, then seep into the air for your child to inhale. If you absolutely can't quit smoking, you can reduce your child's health risks from second-hand smoke considerably by at least smoking outside. Still, even the message that sends is harmful. A past president of the American Heart Association who lives in the heart of tobacco country told me how, during his morning commute, he's shocked to see women in their cars driving their kids to school and simultaneously smoking. The kids are securely strapped in their car seats, but their mom has her window rolled down, cigarette in hand.

Tips for Quitting Smoking

If you really want to quit smoking, you've got to prepare yourself for the often bumpy road ahead. Nicotine addiction can be tough to beat, but with a little troubleshooting, you can do it. Here are the strategies I recommend to my patients:

- Start by picking a specific day to quit, the day you become a nonsmoker.
- Prepare by letting people know you're quitting and surrounding yourself with supportive friends, family members and other nonsmokers. They'll help make you accountable and urge you on. "Hearing everyone tell me they were so glad I was quitting and that they were sure I could do it made me want to quit even more," said Fred, a patient who quit smoking after thirty years of lighting up.
- Keep reminding yourself of the reasons you're quitting. You may want to use visual reminders, such as notes on mirrors or the fridge, or a photo of your kids, to keep you on your game.
- Purge the paraphernalia. Throw away any smoking cues (ashtrays, matches, lighters).
- Steer clear of situations or places that tempt you to smoke, such as bars.

- Talk to your doctor about medical options that can help you quit (nicotine patches, medications and therapy).
- Don't be too hard on yourself. Quitting isn't easy, and if it takes more than one shot, that's okay. If you can't quit the first time, keep trying. Even if you don't succeed right away, consider it practice for when you do.

❏ 5. Keep Your Cholesterol in Check

Cholesterol is a waxy substance that insulates nerves, makes cell membranes and produces certain hormones. However, too much cholesterol plays a large role in determining your risk for CVD. The liver produces all the cholesterol your body needs to function. However, we can take in more cholesterol through diet. Dietary cholesterol is found in animal products such as meat, eggs and dairy. Foods from plants (fruits, vegetables and grains) don't contain any dietary cholesterol and are great substitutes for the above foods.

The "good" cholesterol (HDL, remember H is for *healthy* and we want it *higher*) protects against plaque buildup in your arteries by carrying cholesterol away from the cells and back to the liver for removal from the body. Higher HDL is associated with lower risk for CVD. Too much "bad" cholesterol (LDL, remember L is for *lousy* and we want it *lower*) can cause a buildup of plaque, cholesterol and fat inside walls of the arteries. This condition is called atherosclerosis and can block blood flow to the heart muscle, causing chest pain and increasing your risk for CVD.

Triglycerides (TG) are a form of fat in the blood that comes from the body's fat stores or from the food we eat. Elevated levels can result from consuming too much sugar, alcohol or fat, as well as from having diabetes or being overweight. Often people with high triglyceride levels also have high LDL and low HDL, increasing their risk for heart disease.

Total cholesterol (TC) is HDL cholesterol plus LDL cholesterol and a fraction of triglycerides. This is probably the number you're most familiar with and the number that's often given when visiting a physician. Sometimes your doctor will give you the ratio of your total cholesterol to HDL-cholesterol because this is a good predictor of CVD (should be less than 5 and even lower is better.).

However, it is important to know the cholesterol subtypes because that's what we use when making treatment decisions. Even if your cholesterol isn't abnormal, you can always benefit from watching what you eat, maintaining a healthful diet and getting your cholesterol checked on a regular basis. If you have a genetic cause of high blood cholesterol and/or have premature heart disease in your family, your children (and grandchildren, if applicable) should also have their cholesterol checked after age two.

Your Cholesterol Goals

- Total cholesterol (TC)—less than 200.
- HDL—greater than 50 for women and greater than 40 for men.
- LDL—less than 100; national guidelines suggest that for high-risk patients, including those with a history of CVD and diabetes, an LDL of less than 70 may be a more appropriate goal, based on results of recent studies.
- Triglycerides (TG)—less than 150.

Scoring Your Health Goals

As I've noticed with many of my patients, knowing your cholesterol goals can motivate you to take action. One patient who comes to mind is Lucy, a fifty-seven-year-old pediatric nurse. After learning that her LDL cholesterol was dangerously high, she began eating leaner and, as she puts it, "exercising fiercely." She was able to do this because she was already in pretty good shape because she was on her feet all day as part of her job. After six months, Lucy had lost sixteen pounds, and her cholesterol had dropped over 50 points. "I'm now training for a half marathon," she reported.

For certain people, however, lifestyle change doesn't quite cut it. Medications are recommended to help improve cholesterol levels. Statins, widely used lipid-lowering drugs (lipids are a type of fat produced by your body), are generally prescribed for those with CVD and others with an LDL level above the recommended goal. Keep in mind that these medications don't work alone to lower your cholesterol. You'll still need to pay attention to your diet and exercise and not smoke. To give you an example, I had one patient, Suzanne, who was sixty-one when she was diagnosed with high cholesterol. She exercised, ate right and didn't smoke, but she still ended up with two major and several moderate blockages in her arteries. After undergoing double bypass surgery and finding the right lipid-lowering medication, her cholesterol dropped over 100 points. She hasn't slacked off. "I still maintain a heart-healthy lifestyle because I believe my life of regular exercise before surgery was the one major factor that allowed my heart to continue fighting against my high cholesterol," she said. "If I hadn't been doing that, I don't know where I'd be today."

Many high-risk patients also need medication to improve their HDL and/or triglyceride levels. My dad was told that his "cholesterol" was normal, but it was because his "good" cholesterol was low. In high-risk patients like this, a statin is often combined with niacin or a fibrate to optimize the lipid profile.

It's important to take medications as directed, while also making positive lifestyle changes to lower your cholesterol, such as adopting a heart-healthy diet and getting regular exercise. For more about cholesterol-lowering drugs, see chapter 8.

❏ 6. Keep Tabs on Your Triglycerides

Triglycerides are a form of fat found in food, fat tissue and blood. High levels (greater than 150) are tied to diabetes, obesity and heart disease and can result from consuming too much sugar, alcohol or fats, as well as starches, saturated fat and cholesterol. Good levels come from being at a healthy weight, getting regular exercise and eating a diet low in saturated fat. Eating fish that's rich in omega-3 fatty acids (lake trout, herring, sardines, albacore tuna and salmon) can also help.

❏ 7. Test Your Blood Pressure

Approximately fifty million Americans have high blood pressure, but because the condition usually doesn't have any symptoms, about a third of them don't even know they have it. It's a major risk for CVD. For many of us, getting our blood pressure checked requires a trip to the doctor's office. I recommend getting yours checked at least once a year. But if your blood pressure is on the high side, your doctor may ask you to test your blood pressure at home more often. One of the easiest ways to do that is by purchasing a digital monitor, which takes less than a minute to get an accurate reading. There are three basic types: a manual inflation monitor, which requires you to expand an arm cuff by squeezing a bulb; an automatic inflation monitor with an arm cuff that inflates and deflates at the push of a button; or a wrist monitor, which measures blood pressure and your pulse from the wrist, although blood pressure measurements may not be as accurate those of upper-arm monitors. Ask your doctor about which one is right for you and how often you should check your blood pressure yourself.

Blood pressure is the force created by the heart as it pushes blood into the arteries. Everyone has blood pressure. You need it to live. Each time the heart beats, blood is pumped in and out and creates a surge of pressure in the arteries. This is called systolic (or upper) pressure. When the heart relaxes between beats, the blood pressure goes down, and this is called the diastolic (or lower) pressure. Blood pressure is recorded as these two numbers: systolic/ diastolic. (For example: 118/78, read as "118 over 78.")

Your goal should be to achieve and maintain a blood pressure of less than 120/80 unless instructed otherwise by your doctor. If your blood pressure is 140/90 or greater, you're at higher risk for CVD and other medical problems. Blood pressure between 120/80 and 140/90, or "prehypertension," signals that you don't have high blood pressure yet, but you're likely to develop it unless you adopt the healthful lifestyle changes I'll highlight in this chapter and throughout this book. What's your blood pressure? One in four Americans have high blood pressure; one in two Americans with high blood pressure also suffers from high cholesterol. If you have both, your chance of CVD increases more than just simply adding the two risks together.

> ## THE NEW MATH: 1 + 1 = 3
>
> When you have two major CVD risk factors, such as high blood pressure and high cholesterol, your risk of heart attack may be greater than just the two combined. It's important to pay attention and treat both. The good news is that the benefits of treatment are usually greatest among those with multiple risk factors.

A Note from Dr. Lori: Kids and Blood Pressure

Recent studies show that as many as two million American children and teens have high blood pressure. Poor diet, lack of exercise and obesity may be to blame. The consequences of unmanaged hypertension in children includes enlarged hearts, kidney problems, a thickening of part of the blood vessels that may cause hardening of the arteries and being at even greater risk for high blood pressure as an adult. The tendency for high blood pressure can be inherited from one or both parents, which is why I urge my patients with high blood pressure to have their childrens' blood pressure checked as well. The American Heart Association recommends that children age three and older have their blood pressure checked yearly. Is your child at risk? Find out by getting their blood pressure checked at their next doctor's visit.

❏ 8. Derail Diabetes

Once you have diabetes, you always have a higher risk of CVD than those who don't have diabetes. But there's still a lot you can do to lower your chances of a heart attack or stroke. Many of my patients have diabetes, and I always stress to them how important it is to maintain tight control of their blood glucose while research determines how tight is best for the heart. Overall, your goal should be to keep your HbA1c (a measure of your average glucose control over a span of three months) at less than 7 percent and a fasting glucose at less than 100 mg/dL (or nonfasting glucose at less than 140 mg/dL). You also need to keep an especially close watch on your blood pressure, cholesterol and BMI. A national study of those with diabetes shows that as weight goes up, so does the risk for developing CVD.

To do all this, you'll need to work closely with your health care team. For the patients I see with diabetes, I'm typically one of several health care providers on their team. One of my patients, Cathy, who is forty-six, for example, also sees a diabetes nutrition educator, an endocrinologist and a primary care physician. "But it's worth it because I feel like my diabetes doesn't have to be a death sentence." And she has plenty of reason to live, with two kids in middle school!

If you don't have diabetes, do what you can to prevent it. The good news: many of the lifestyle habits that help prevent heart disease also help reduce your risk of diabetes, so you'll get a two-for-one. And a recent major study showed lifestyle improvements were even more effective than medication in preventing the onset of diabetes. Get your blood glucose tested, especially if you have a BMI of 25 or more.

❏ 9. Manage Your Mental Health

Watch for signs of depression, and get treatment if you need it. I'll talk about depression in the next chapter, as well as other psychological factors that affect CVD risk, such as stress, social isolation, anger and anxiety. I'm a firm believer in the mind-body connection. When I get stressed (work, the kids, too much to do) exercise is key for my stress management, so by exercising every-day I get to check two things off my list (I talk more about stress management in chapter 4).

Time for a Checkup?

To keep track of your blood pressure and blood cholesterol, get regular checkups starting at age twenty. As I mentioned in chapter 2, I get a checkup every year around my birthday—my present to myself. When you think about it, we start off our lives with well-baby checkups. I think it's important to carry on that tradition throughout our lives because we know that if we can catch some-thing early there's a much greater likelihood of fixing it. Plus, as I mentioned, getting regular checkups allows you to establish a rela-tionship with your doctor so that when you have symptoms, you have someone to call with whom you're comfortable. So many of my patients tell me how they've avoided calling or going to a doctor, and I think it was often because they didn't have a rapport with one. Instead, many waited until they couldn't wait any longer and showed up in the emergency room. Each year in your calen-dar, on your birthday month, write, "Make doctor's appointment for a checkup." Then do it.

DR. LORI'S CHECKUP CHECKLIST

Not all checkups are alike. Here's a checklist to make sure yours gives you the information you need to monitor your health status. Here's a baseline of what needs to be checked:

❏ Blood cholesterol. To get accurate blood cholesterol results—we're talking LDL, HDL, triglycerides and total cholesterol—you'll need to fast, typically for nine to twelve hours before your cholesterol test. That means no eating or drinking, other than water, after midnight. If you're not medically able to fast, only your total and HDL cholesterol should be done.
❏ Blood pressure.
❏ Blood glucose.
❏ Weight.
❏ Waist circumference.
❏ BMI.

Use the following chart to track your weight/BMI, waist circumference, cholesterol, blood pressure and blood sugar. Feel free to photocopy it and pass it around to your spouse/partner and your parents. Keep one for each of your kids (get their ideal numbers from your doctor). These are the important numbers to track. Use them to monitor your health and stay motivated to live well for yourself and those who care about you. Consider keeping a copy and carrying it around in your purse or wallet, like you would a credit card, so you'll always be in the know.

Risk Factor Tracker

Date					
Weight Goal: BMI between 18.5–24.9					
Weight Circumference Goal: Less than 35 inches (women); Less than 40 inches (men)					
Total Cholesterol Goal: Less than 200					
LDL Goal: Less than 100					
HDL Goal: Greater than 50 (women); greater than 40 (men)					
Triglycerides Goal: Less than 150					
Blood Pressure Goal: Less than 120/80 (ideally)					
HbA1c or Nonfasting Glucose Goal: HbA1c less than 7 percent; fasting glucose less than 100 (or nonfasting glucose less than 140)					

Peering into the Crystal Ball

To recap, you're at increased risk for CVD if you smoke, have hypertension, low HDL levels, high LDL levels, a family history of premature CVD, or are age forty-five or older (men) or age fifty-five or older (women). But to get an even clearer idea of your risk for CVD, log on to *http://www.nhlbi.nih.gov/guidelines/cholesterol/index.htm* and click on the "10-year Risk Calculator for Patients." This online risk-assessment tool uses information from the renowned Framingham Heart Study to calculate a person's chances of having a heart attack or dying of heart disease in the next ten years. The tool is designed for adults between ages twenty and seventy-nine who don't have CVD or diabetes.

To calculate your risk (and those of family members), you'll need to input age, gender, total cholesterol number, HDL cholesterol and your systolic blood pressure (the first number in your blood pressure reading). You'll also need to answer yes or no to whether you're currently on medication to treat high blood pressure or you smoke.

In general, you're at high risk for CVD if the score calculated is greater than 20 percent. You're at intermediate risk if your score is 10 to 20 percent. You're at lower risk of having a heart attack in the next ten years if your score is less than 10 percent. The score you receive can help you and your doctor determine the right CVD treatment plan for you, based on your gender. One caveat is that some people who score in the low-risk group are actually intermediate risk if they have a very high level of a single risk factor, such as cholesterol (indicating a genetic problem) or if they have a family history of premature heart disease or if there is evidence of what we call "subclinical" disease, such as calcium deposits on a coronary scan.

Preventive Guidelines for Women

Beginning in the 1950s, it was common for women to be advised by the media on how to take care of their husband's hearts, with no mention of their own. That tactic hit home when I was in college, and the father of a very good friend of mine had heart disease and needed bypass surgery. During the father's recovery, my friend's mother took over all of the household chores, including snow shoveling, which was a big job because the family lived in Vermont. One day, when she was out clearing the driveway, she dropped dead of a stroke (a form of CVD). It's a classic example of how, as women, we're often taking care of everyone else instead of ourselves. But we shouldn't forget that we also need to be tended to because CVD doesn't spare either gender. In fact, over the past twenty years, CVD has killed more women than men in the United States. During that time, the CVD death rate has declined significantly for men but remained constant for women. Fortunately, times have changed dramatically, and we're now much more aware of women's CVD risk.

To help improve the outlook for women, in February 2004 the American Heart Association issued the first set of comprehensive, evidence-based guidelines for the prevention of CVD in women. I was privileged to serve as chair of the expert panel that wrote the guidelines and included representatives from a dozen professional and government organizations, and I can say without hesitation that this was a landmark collaborative initiative. The guidelines emphasize how important it is to assess the future heart disease risk and categorize women as high, intermediate or lower risk to help determine the intensity of preventive therapy. Although the guidelines are designed to help your doctor recommend a preventive treatment plan, you should also know your own risk and discuss it with your doctor. In general, here are the preventive strategies we recommend for women, depending on their risk category.

WOMEN'S CVD PREVENTION GUIDELINES

All Women	Regular exercise, not smoking, eating a heart-healthy diet and maintaining a healthy weight.

Women at low risk (less than 10 percent risk of having a heart attack in the next ten years)	• Don't take aspirin for heart disease prevention. If you are over sixty-five, discuss possible stroke benefits as well as possible bleeding side effects with your doctor.
	• Ask your doctor about taking:
	  —a cholestrol-lowering drug if your LDL level is greater than or = to 190 or if you have risk factors for CVD and your LDL is greater than or = to 160.
	  —prescription niacin or fibrate therapy if your HDL level is low or your triglyceride level is high after your LDL goal is reached.
	• Ask your doctor about drugs to lower blood pressure if you are above 140/90, or even lower if you have diabetes.

Women at intermediate risk (10 to 20 percent risk of heart attack within the next ten years)	• Ask your doctor about taking: —aspirin if your blood pressure is under control and you're at low risk of gastrointestinal bleeding or bleeding type of stroke. —a cholesterol-lowering drug if your LDL levels are greater than or = 130. —prescription niacin or a fibrate drug if your HDL level is low or your tiglyceride level is high after LDL goal is reached. • Ask your doctor about drugs to lower your blood pressure if you are above 140/90, or even lower if you have diabetes.
Women at high risk (greater than 20 percent risk of having a heart attack in the next ten years)	• Ask your doctor about taking: —aspirin or another clot inhibitor. —a statin (even if your LDL is below 100). —prescription niacin or a fibrate drug if your HDL level is low or your triglyceride level is high. —an angiotensin-converting enzyme (ACE) inhibitor or angiotensin-receptor blocker (ARB) if you can't take an ACE inhibitor. —a beta-blocker if you have had a heart attack or have symptomatic heart disease. • Seek an evaluation and treatment for depression if you suspect you may be clinically depressed. (For more on depression and CVD, see chapter 4.)

I take these guidelines to heart for my female patients, myself and my own mother, who has high blood pressure. She's a prime example of someone who takes care of everyone else ahead of herself. Only recently have we begun to seriously discuss her blood pressure and how to manage it. It took a lot from both of us. She didn't want to bother me because she thought I was busy enough already, and I, well, I don't think I wanted to admit that Mom, someone who worked, raised five kids, kept a neat house, canned her own tomatoes, made her own sauce and helped take care of my father after his heart attack, wasn't invincible. That can be a tough realization for any child, even if you're a doctor. So, Mom, how is your blood pressure? These guidelines helped us to start talking. I hope this book will help you broach the subject of blood pressure, and CVD in general, with your loved one too.

A NOTE FROM DR. LORI: WHAT'S YOUR RISK?

Less than 10 percent of women are at an optimal risk level for heart disease. What's your risk level? Finding out is your first step to reducing the great divide between your knowledge and your actions.

Beating Bad Genes

Does heart disease lurk in your family history? Not sure? Find out! The following guidelines can help you get an accurate glimpse of your family medical history so you can alert and work with your doctor to develop a CVD prevention plan of attack.

To trace your family medical history, the first step is making a list or drawing a picture of your family tree. For help, log on to *www.hhs.gov/familyhistory,* a government site that can help you catalog the information to give your doctor a head start in calculating your disease risk. Go as far back as your great-grandparents, if you can, and record, for each family member, who had what particular condition and how old they were when they were diagnosed and/or died from it. Include cousins, aunts and uncles if you can. Be on the lookout for heart attacks as well as any vascular disease, such as stroke, arterial disease of the legs or an abdominal aneurysm (a swelling in the wall of the largest artery in the abdomen), because these conditions increase your risk for CVD. As I mentioned, if you have a first-degree relative who had a heart attack or vascular disease prematurely (younger than age sixty-five for women and age fifty-five for men), you're especially vulnerable, not only because of shared genes but, if you lived with that family member, shared lifestyle as well, which may be just as important. Your cholesterol level comes from food and your family.

Past generations weren't as open about their medical problems as we are today. If a relative died of cancer, for example, it was common not even to say the word, but rather to say the family member simply "got sick" or died of "old age." But in truth, we all die of something much more specific than that. To get answers and fill in the blanks of your family medical history, you may have to ask pointed questions and do a bit of digging. Your family may be reluctant to talk about it, but press on. I've had adopted patients who tracked down medical information about their biological family members—they were that motivated. But the legwork is worth it because the information you gather may save your life and your children's.

Talk with your primary care physician about any disease or condition you're concerned about that's highlighted in your family medical tree. Any heart disease in your family? Studies have shown that only about 30 percent of physicians take a proper family history, so it's up to you to lay the groundwork for them. The specific information you provide may change the way they manage your health care. Remember, be sure to mention any vascular problems in the family—from heart disease and stroke to retinal disease or blood vessel problems in the lower legs.

Stay Current and Compliant

Once you've been prescribed a preventive or treatment regimen, stay up to date by doing your own research, and take your medication as prescribed. I'll discuss medication compliance in more detail in chapter 8. The Internet can be an excellent source of information if you log on to reputable Web sites, such as *www.american heart.org,* the Web site for the American Heart Association. Our preventive cardiology team at NewYork-Presbyterian Hospital also updates information consistent with national prevention guidelines on a regular basis, so please pay us a visit at *www.heart healthtimes.com.* Also, be sure to check in with your doctor regularly to make sure your regimen is in keeping with current recommendations. Keep asking your primary care physician or specialist, "Is there anything new in this field?" Treatments, therapies and screening measures for CVD can change significantly in just a few years. As a doctor, I know it's okay to ask! Refer back to chapter 2 for more on how to work with your doctor.

Testing, Testing, Testing

Besides tracking the traditional risk factors for gauging CVD risk, such as measuring blood cholesterol and blood pressure, researchers have discovered several "novel" markers that may also signal you're a target for CVD. They include C-reactive protein (CRP), homocysteine, LDL particle number and lipoprotein (a). Maybe you've heard about them; they seem to be constantly in the news.

CRP is a compound in the blood that's produced in the liver in response to infection or trama from something as fleeting as a sore throat to something more chronic, such as rheumatoid arthritis. There appears to be a strong link between low-grade inflammation, as reflected by elevated levels of high sensitivity CRP, or hsCRP, in the blood and CVD. Elevated levels of hsCRP can predict the risk of CVD in apparently healthy men and women, as well as among those with CVD. In fact, I've had patients referred to me who had "normal" cholesterol, but ended up with a heart attack. When I went back to investigate what went wrong, I discovered that some of them had high CRP. Although studies have shown CRP helps predict CVD, we don't know for sure that lowering it by itself reduces risk. Because of this, many doctors don't routinely measure this or other novel risk factors.

Homocysteine is an amino acid (also a protein) in the blood that may promote the buildup of fatty deposits in your arteries by damaging the inner lining of arteries and promoting blood clots. Too much homocysteine is correlated with an increased risk of CVD. Folic acid can lower levels of homocysteine, but data are inconsistent on whether it protects the heart, and for patients with recent angioplasty, it could make things worse.

Lipoprotein (a)—Lp(a)—is a fatty protein substance in the blood that resembles LDL cholesterol. Elevated levels—more than 30 mg/dL—are believed to increase the risk of CVD twofold in whites but not blacks. Roughly 1/3 of patients with pre-mature heart disease have elevated levels of Lp(a.). Although Lp(a) may be a risk factor for CVD, research is not available to prove that lowering Lp(a) lowers CVD risk.

Should You Worry About Novel Risk Factors?

In my opinion, it's too soon to tell because we just don't know yet whether treating these "numbers" translates to fewer heart attacks. Treating other risk factors, such as high cholesterol and high blood pressure, which are tried-and-true approaches, should be the primary focus in practice. In any event, if you're concerned, ask your doctor whether you'll benefit from having hsCRP testing, or any one of these additional blood tests. With my patients, I tend to do these tests when I'm really on the fence about whether to give someone a statin or recommend an even more aggressive preventive treatment plan. In general, I don't perform a test unless the information I gain from it changes how I'll manage a condition. And because there is such a thing as a false positive, I don't want to concern my patients unnecessarily.

One patient of mine, who was among what I call "the worried well," insisted on having his C-reactive protein checked every month because he was convinced that this test was going to indicate whether he was going to have a heart attack. But as I mentioned, C-reactive protein can rise as a result of any inflammation in the body, even something as small as a blister on your foot. So you can see how easy it could be to become misled by this test. I finally had to say to this patient, "It's great that you're interested in your health and your risk factors. But there needs to be a healthy balance between knowing enough and not worrying too much."

Ways to Spy on Your Arteries

If you're at high risk for CVD, your doctor may order a stress test, sometimes called a treadmill test, to determine how well your heart is working. During the test, you're hooked up to equipment that monitors the heart. At first, you walk slowly on the treadmill, and then the pace picks up, and the treadmill is tilted to mimic a small hill. You may be asked to breathe into a tube for a couple of minutes. Afterward, you sit or lie down and have your heart and blood pressure checked.

If a stress test indicates that something's up, your doctor may order a more sophisticated stress test (combined with a nuclear scan or echocardiogram). Sometimes the doctor will order the more sophisticated test first because you may have electrical abnormalities of the heart that make it difficult to interpret a regular stress test. And sometimes a medicine that increases your heart rate will be given instead of running on a treadmill if you have orthopedic problems that preclude the standard test.

If your stress test is abnormal and your doctor is suspicious, he or she may order an angiogram, an invasive test that can detect whether your arteries are, in fact, clogged. To perform an angiogram, a thin tube (catheter) is inserted into an artery and threaded up to the heart, after which a special fluid goes through the catheter to allow the arteries to show up well on X-ray.

Newer tests are on the horizon, though, that are much less invasive, but these are still considered "for research only." They are quicker and less invasive, but the angiogram is still considered our "gold standard" for diagnosing heart disease.

A computerized tomography (CT) scan of the arteries, which measures calcium buildup, is another diagnostic technique that shows promise. Calcium in the walls of coronary arteries (coronary artery calcium or CAC) is a sign of atherosclerosis or clogged arteries. Still, like novel risk factors, we don't yet know if this test substantially improves the predictability of CVD over traditional tests, such as measuring cholesterol and other risk factors. Your doctor can tell you whether a CAC scan or any one of the newer technologies is right for you. I tend to consider these tests for patients who have a family history of heart disease but don't have traditional risk factors for CVD, such as high LDL or low HDL cholesterol.

Managing Blood Pressure

High blood pressure, often called hypertension, is referred to as "the silent killer" because it doesn't usually cause any symptoms. In fact, you can look and feel fine while having very high blood pressure and being at high risk for CVD. Anyone can have high blood pressure. Those who are overweight, smoke or have a family history of hypertension are at higher risk for high blood pressure. Find out if you have high blood pressure by getting your blood pressure checked regularly, and then take the appropriate steps to lower it if it's high. If it's normal, that's great. Learn how to keep it that way. We'll talk more about this in the following chapters.

The Fifty-Thousand-Mile Checkup

We all go through hormonal changes throughout our lives, but there are two points when our hormones undergo dramatic changes. One of them is puberty and, for women, the other is menopause. I used to kid my son Matt when he was fourteen to be as patient with me when I go through menopause as I tried to be with him in puberty. In fact, my husband and I coined the term "Mattopause" to describe this transition in life. With menopause, which is the second significant hormonal milestone in a woman's life (and probably a man's as well!), the ovaries gradually stop producing estrogen. What's surprising to many of my female patients is how insidious the reulting symptoms can be. Symptoms can actually start in your early forties, and you may not even realize they're premenopausal signs. You may have just a little bit more trouble sleeping, or you can't quite grab the name of that person. Maybe you're moodier than usual or even have a few hot flashes or night sweats. Then, as you get closer to actual menopause, the average age of which is fifty-one, night sweats and hot flashes can worsen.

At menopause, I like women to come in for what I call the fifty-thousand-mile checkup because that's when many risk factors worsen in women. Hormone replacement therapy (HRT) hasn't been shown to prevent CVD, and in some women it may actually increase risk. Still, menopause is a critical time to discuss your options for risk-factor control. If you decide to try HRT to help alleviate menopausal symptoms, talk to your doctor about taking it at the lowest dose for the shortest duration possible, such as one to one and a half years, then tapering it off gradually.

It's fascinating to me how many women come in at age fifty at their own intuitive urging. Often, they're not the cheeriest of patients. Fueled by menopause, they may be teary eyed. Their kids are gone, they choke. Some claim they're fat and ugly and useless to their husbands. They've come to me to get their act together—fast. But they don't know where to begin because it has been so long since they've focused on themselves. It's hard to undo twenty years of neglect. Some women can pull themselves out of it and put themselves at the top of their "to-do" lists, which I'll discuss in detail in chapter 7, but I encourage you not to put yourself in that position.

If you're in your twenties, thirties or forties, and you notice that your weight starts to creep up (five pounds is a red flag), take that as a warning sign that you need to pay more attention to yourself.

A weekly weigh-in can help you monitor your situation. If you notice an upward trend on the scale, ask yourself what you've been doing lately that might have caused it, then fine-tune your weight-loss or weight-maintenance efforts. We'll cover weight loss in an upcoming chapter.

All told, it's best to develop good habits in your twenties, thirties and forties through heart-healthy living to prevent weight gain in the first place. As many of my patients can attest, it's so much easier to prevent weight gain than it is to lose weight once the pounds have found a home. Still, it can be done. "The key is to clarify your goals," says Rosemarie, a fifty-four-year-old patient of mine who lost forty pounds in two years by exercising at least half an hour every day, eating more fruits, vegetables, grains and fish, and eating fewer high-fat foods. In turn, she reached healthy cholesterol and blood pressure levels. "At the rate I was going, I owed it to myself to take action," she said.

Three Keys to Your Heart

Here are three key points I hope you'll take to heart from this chapter:

1. **Make lifestyle your top priority.** Eat well, exercise, lose weight if you're overweight and don't smoke. Even if you have normal cholesterol levels, you're not off the hook. What we eat affects our hearts apart from cholesterol. And all the exercise in the world can't undo a bad diet.

2. **Know your numbers.** Most Americans don't know their cholesterol levels and other risk factors, even though they understand, for example, that high cholesterol is bad for them. But how can you lower your risk if you don't know what it is? Record your numbers in the "Risk Factor Tracker" and have them with you—in your purse or wallet—so you can discuss your progress when you see your doctor. Keeping track of your numbers will help prevent them from slowly creeping up on you.

3. **Tell your doctor if you have heart disease or any vascular disease in your family.** This is especially important if any of your immediate family members (mother, father or sibling) are diagnosed with CVD before fifty-five (men) or sixty-five (women). Your doctor needs to know so he or she can screen and work with you to tailor a preventive action plan that's personally designed to lower your CVD risk and improve your health. Remember, your family history doesn't have to be your destiny. Most major risk can be managed through lifestyle and medication when necessary.

Chapter

Find Your Inner Sanctuary

"The soul is a garden enclosed, our own perpetual paradise where we can be refreshed and restored."

—Thomas Moore

It's so easy for me to write prescriptions and so much harder to practice medicine. It takes time and tenderness to deal with the root causes of CVD. They're complicated because they include psychological factors such as stress, worry, depression, anger, isolation, denial and anxiety, which often lead to poor lifestyle habits that then lead to high blood pressure, abnormal cholesterol and diabetes. To make matters worse, psychological factors may have a direct affect on disease risk as well. All the prescriptions in the world can't overcome the damaging effects of these emotions. In fact, in a study called INTERHEART conducted in fifty-two countries that involved almost twenty-five thousand people, those who suffered a heart attack were 45 percent more likely to report several periods of stress at work or home in the preceding twelve months. Traumatic life events such as separation or divorce and depression were also much more common in those individuals who developed heart disease.

Our heart acts as a kind of a psychological barometer. If you find yourself in the path of an oncoming bus, your heart pounds with fear. If you get interrupted by a telemarketer at dinnertime, your blood pressure boils with irritation and anger. Even now we're just learning how a chronic, daily dose of such negative emotions affects our long-term heart health. Based on the compelling body of evidence, I am convinced they are bona fide risk factors all by themselves.

I would not have been such a believer if I had not had a patient, Gerald, prove that point. Gerald was a high-ranking politician who came to me for CVD prevention. Gerald had such a stressful life, he explained, because he was constantly working 'round the clock, putting out fires, glad-handing constituents and participating in government committees. "I just want to make sure I'm okay" he spewed in staccato sound bites as he reached to answer his cell phone.

Ironically, I thought Gerald was a member of what I call the "worried well" because, frankly, I couldn't find anything particularly alarming about his risk assessment. In his early forties, Gerald had no impressive CVD risk factors. His cholesterol and his blood pressure were relatively good. He was thin and exercised every day. He was also a vegetarian, so his diet was probably low in saturated fat. Still, Gerald not only talked fast, he thought and moved quickly as he peppered me with question after question. It was obvious to me that Gerald's mind was on overdrive. What could I say to this overachieving patient? "Your personality is your risk factor," I finally concluded. "You just need to slow down, relax, enjoy your life. Find some pleasure. Don't worry so much. You're literally going to worry yourself to death."

Oh, how I wish my warning hadn't turned out to be foretelling. Two years after Gerald visited my office, his wife called, informing me that Gerald had, in fact, suffered a fatal heart attack. I'll never forget how shocked I was for days, weeks and months afterward.

Gerald just didn't fit the traditional profile of a heart attack candidate. When one of my patients dies of a heart attack, it is a personal failure for me as a specialist in preventive cardiology because my life's work is to stop people from having them. It was also tough to take because, besides his wife, Gerald had left an eight-year-old daughter behind—and neither had had the chance to say good-bye.

It was a poignant personal lesson. In retrospect, I think I should have been firmer with Gerald, and yes, lectured him about how chronic stress really *can* kill you. On some level, I think he knew he needed to take his foot off the accelerator. There are so many patients like Gerald who are never confronted because it's too difficult a conversation to have—especially in an environment that requires many physicians to see X patients per hour. Sometimes doctors just don't want to confront issues that are important but uncomfortable for patients to address. But now, when Geraldesque patients come to my office, I talk openly about this soft area of medicine. I ask them why they need to do so much. Often, I suspect these patients feel a loss of control, that if they do not keep on top of things their lives will get away from them. Ironically, they appear powerful and in control, but inside there is a very real and quiet desperation.

A year after Gerald died, his wife graciously called me again, saying she just wanted to let me know that she and her daughter were doing okay and that she was running for her husband's political seat. "Our daughter is helping with the campaign," she said proudly. I thought, *That's amazing how life goes on.* They were able to rebound from this tragic event and carry on his work. Still, I fought back the tears as I heard the update. Overall, I've learned not to hold back anymore when I meet patients who are in the process of self-destructing, because I know their lives and the happiness of their families are on the line.

Minding Matters of the Heart

Although it may seem relatively new, researchers have been examining the role psychological factors play in preventing heart disease for nearly half a century. In the late 1950s, some of the earliest research linked stress, such as the loss of a job or loved one, with the increased risk of CVD. Through the years, scientists have found that certain adverse psychological factors, such as depression, social isolation, chronic anger and certain kinds of anxiety, affect both your behavior and your health. Hostility and anger have long been suspected of being major players in CVD. Free-floating or easily aroused anger, in fact, is one of the two symptoms of type A behavior (the other being time pressure). Type A behavior was one of the first psychological conditions suggested as a risk factor for CVD.

There are many ways in which psychological factors are related to CVD. It's suggested that people with adverse psychological factors (stress, anger, depression and anxiety, for example) may be more likely to have an unhealthful lifestyle. They may overeat, not exercise, smoke or smoke more, or drink too much and avoid exercising to cope with negative feelings. One patient of mine, for example, Sherry, a television producer in her early fifties, was relying on little more than caffeine and adrenaline to propel her through the day. I had to convince her that food was her friend, especially fruits and vegetables, whole grains, fish and low-fat dairy products. To help her stay committed to her new, more healthful eating style, she began keeping a food diary. "I also start my day by taking five 'mental minutes' to visualize what's likely to derail my best intentions," she said. Lifestyle factors, such as diet and exercise, can mediate the relationship between stress and heart disease risk. She was working to prevent stress—which is what everyone should do.

In addition, excess chronic overstimulation of th[e] nervous system—the "fight or flight" response—may physiological changes that promote atheroscleros[is] buildup of plaque deposits in the arteries of the heart. During fight or flight, your sympathetic nervous system revs up and your heart gallops. Your palms sweat; your breathing becomes shallow. The message: Your personal safety is threatened. Danger! Get out of the way! Fight or flight is helpful if you need to flee from an attacker or move out of the way of an oncoming bus. But it can be damaging, even deadly, when it gets stuck "on" and you're only trying to, for example, eliminate the piles in your inbox or cross ten things off your to-do list by 5 P.M. It's important to recognize symptoms of stress just as it is important to know symptoms of a heart attack. Signs of stress may include:

- Feeling irritable
- Difficulty sleeping
- Over- or undereating
- Difficulty concentrating
- Abusing drugs or alcohol
- Feeling anxious
- Gaining or losing excessive amounts of weight
- Feeling overwhelmed at home or work

Women, especially, may have both professional and domestic responsibilities that can lead to an increased level of stress. You may be caring for others and sometimes neglect your own needs or put others before yourself—the oxygen-mask syndrome I discuss in chapter 7. Stress may produce negative effects on your body by increasing blood pressure and heart rate and by constricting coronary blood vessels. In those who already have arterial plaque, studies show that both chronic stress and acute stress from major, catastrophic events, such as an earthquake or

September 11, can also spark plaque rupture in the blood vessels, which can then cause fatal heart attacks, arrhythmias and nonfatal heart attacks. Both may also cause significant cardiac abnormalities, such as myocardial ischemia, a condition in which the heart doesn't get enough blood.

After the World Trade Center disaster, my preventive-cardiology team at NewYork-Presbyterian Hospital established a heart attack prevention program and found that many people were suffering symptoms of heart disease and didn't know it. We also found at four months and at one year later, many of the victims and family members we screened had adopted behaviors in response to the stress, such as staying inside, not exercising, smoking and eating more than usual, which could increase their long-term heart disease risk.

Fortunately, there are ways to keep stress from getting the best of you. Here's what I suggest (and live by) for keeping your cool— and your heart healthy—when the going gets tough.

Ah, Solitude

One of the most significant ways I think our fast-paced, to-do-list-driven society is getting to us and inciting CVD is our lack of solitude. This isn't to be confused with social isolation, the type of aloneness I referred to earlier as a risk factor. What I'm talking about is downtime, time for ourselves to just think and reflect and call our own.

It may sound frivolous, but I believe solitude is critical to our heart health. Think about it. When is the last time you had time to yourself, to ponder and do whatever you wanted, without someone pulling at you, demanding your action or your attention? In my opinion, it's important for our heart health to find space in our lives just for us, to clear our minds and recharge. In fact, I literally write prescriptions for my patients: "Thirty min/day of solitude." During that half hour, "No one is to talk to you, and you are to find a minisanctuary of your own," I instruct them.

Personally, I build solitude into my day by arranging my home with that in mind. In my backyard, for example, I reserve a small patio area that's relatively hidden from view of the neighbors and my family (to find me, they have to come looking). It sports one chair, which is just for me, so that I can sit alone and think. Short on space? No problem. Just take possession of a spot in any room in your home, and designate a chair that is yours. It should face something peaceful, like the glow of a candle or trees, but not the TV.

I also find solitude in everyday tasks, such as cleaning my house. I'm not a big fan of the do-leg-lifts-while-you're-washing-dishes school of thought. In fact, I think solo-tasking is a much more healthful ideal for our hearts and our minds. For me, tidying up is therapeutic. When I'm dusting or straightening up the book-shelf, I'm getting immediate gratification. I get into a zone and lose track of time. If the phone rings, I'm startled. Call me crazy, but I don't perceive housecleaning as something awful I have to do, but as something I really enjoy that's healthful for me. It gets my mind off thinking about the kids, work or what I need to do next. That's why I urge you to take chores—whether it's yard work or vacuuming—and regard them as a way to get some physical activity and much-needed time "in the zone."

Still, if you absolutely abhor cleaning, don't fire your house-keeper. Instead, find something else that works for you. Need more ideas? I have lately been encouraging my patients to place signs on their bathroom doors that say, "Do not disturb for thirty minutes." I tell them to take a bath for a half hour, three times a week, that's infused with essential oils. Aromatherapy, using the fragrances of flower essences, aromatic tree barks and fruit, can help elicit a feeling of inner peace. My favorite is spruce and pine needles because I feel like I am outside in a forest and in harmony with nature. An aromatherapy bath is a perfect way to combine the transformative benefits of scent and the naturally soothing properties of water. Basic essential oils that can turn a bath into a "scent-sational" experience include peppermint, spearmint, spruce, pine, orange blossom, ylang ylang, lavender and sandalwood. Experiment. Aromatherapy baths are one of my personal favorite ways to unwind because I can tailor scents to my needs and cherish my time alone.

Of course, being at home can be associated with interruptions despite your best intentions. Even though I have my special place to reflect and relax at home, there's no telling when the phone or the doorbell will ring and disrupt it.

When I'm desperate for some solitude because I've really had a challenging week or too much on my plate for too long, I pay a visit to the holistic fitness center in my neighborhood. It's called CGI and has an Eastern philosophy. C is for Korean *chun*, which means heaven, G is for *gi*, which means earth, and I is for *in*, which means human. CGI's purpose is to enhance the harmony between heaven, earth and us. At CGI, they feature "healing" cool and hot aromatherapy baths in special granite tubs. I especially love it because there's no talking allowed and no beepers or cell phones, which is why I chose it over other health clubs. When I go to CGI, I can center myself, find my balance, my inner peace and my place in the bigger universe. If you, too, can find a sanctuary outside your home, whether it's a spa or a nature park, I encourage you to make regular visits to refresh.

Family Downtime

Over the years, my kids have become tuned in to my need for solitude. They'll jokingly pat me on the back and say, "Time to go to CGI, Mom," or, "Can I get the bath ready for you?" And now they've started taking baths themselves as a way to decompress. They're boys at the crest of adolescence, but teens need to escape, too, to center themselves and get away from stimuli, like video games, cell phones, Ipods and instant messaging. In fact, I think it's important that everyone in the family has opportunities for solitude and centering, even preschoolers. It's never too early to teach your kids this life skill.

We invest so much in our children's education by accentuating reading, writing, math and SAT scores. But I believe we need to put equal emphasis on teaching our children how to relax, to develop inner resources they can call upon to calm themselves down in stressful periods. It is not only for their heart health, but also for their general well-being, so they do not turn to alcohol or drugs as a means to escape the stressors of life. Down the road, when my sons are in college, I want them to turn inward, not outward—nor cave in to peer pressure—to cope when the pressure is on. Most kids these days unwind by turning to TV. But that's an outward activity. It's not the same as turning inward and learning how to tune in to yourself.

It's one more thing to have to think about as a parent, I know. But it's important to at least introduce relaxation methods, such as deep breathing, stretching and quiet time, to our kids. Exercise, stretching and deep breathing are great ways for people of all ages to center themselves, but it is best to learn how early.

Bolster Your Support System

Just as it's imperative to have time alone, it's vital for our heart health to have support from others when we need it. Research suggests that having a strong social network, such as being in a close relationship or belonging to one or more organizations such as a church, is associated with a reduced risk of CVD.

Truth is, we know very little about the underlying physiological pathways linking social isolation to increased CVD or mortality in general. Nonetheless, a strong support system seems to have a twofold benefit: It may reduce the physiological impact of stress on the heart; it may also help us take better care of ourselves by influencing the extent to which we engage in healthy behaviors. When we have a good support network, we're less likely to smoke, eat a high-fat diet and consume too much alcohol.

So work to keep the friends you have, especially those who help enable you to live healthfully. Making new friends is not always easy because, well, we are all so busy these days. In fact, when I encourage my patients to try to forge new friendships, they look at me blankly and say, "How?" or, "When?" I can relate. As a wife, mother and busy physician-scientist, I don't have lots of time to make new friends. Anything that would take me away from my kids would likely make me feel more guilt than pleasure anyway. So one thing I do is make friends with the parents of my kids' friends. It's a win/win situation. I enjoy spending time with other parents at my sons' swimming and diving meets and the neighborhood pool, and that makes me feel connected.

One of my favorite events of the year is Family Night Out at our local swim club. The parents enjoy a glass of wine and dinner while the kids play volleyball and dance to a DJ. By the end of the evening, we're all swaying to the music and feeling like we're part of something special that's bigger than ourselves. Maybe there are

opportunities for friendships in your everyday life you can culti-
vate, too. Because the need for belonging is as important to an
adult as it is to a teenager, my advice is to do what you can, and
grow where you're planted.

For some of my patients who may be socially isolated, I recommend considering volunteer work. I tell them it may be as powerful
in reducing their risk of a heart attack or death as the prescriptions
I write them to lower their cholesterol or blood pressure.

A NOTE FROM DR. LORI: FUNCTIONAL SUPPORT

If you already have heart disease, you'll need what's called
functional support to reduce your risk of heart attack.
Functional support means perceiving that you have a close-
knit group of friends or at least one person you can rely on
and confide in, someone with whom you can truly be yourself. That level of perceived emotional support appears to be
critical, especially for patients with CVD.

Keep the Faith

I mentioned church as a source of human connection, and
indeed, one of the ways some of my patients find companionship
is through their religious organizations. The benefits they receive
because of this affiliation and their faith seem to go much deeper
than friendships.

One patient, Helen, comes to mind. In her late sixties, Helen
has many dragons to slay. Not only does she have CVD, but
she's also taking care of a disabled husband and raising her
three-year-old grandson because her daughter is in a mental

institution. She has every reason in the world to be stressed and depressed. Without question, her situation would drive most of us to the brink. Yet Helen is tranquil. My long list of things to do is nothing compared to what Helen deals with daily. It's humbling. "How do you do it?" I finally asked her during one visit. "Helen, how do you get through the day?"

"Dr. Mosca," she said, "I pray, and I know my Lord is going to take care of me," she said. I sincerely believe Helen has thrived as long as she has because of her religion. It seems to center her, comfort her and provide relief.

Prayer can be many things, including a way to feel listened to and supported. When you talk to God, you get the floor. Consider finding a religion or spiritually fulfilling activity that suits you, if you haven't already. You don't necessarily need to join a religious organization to reap these benefits. A spiritual activity could be simply getting involved in something you care about deeply.

Deal with Depression

Each year, according to the National Institute of Mental Health (NIMH), nearly nineteen million Americans ages eighteen and over suffer from some form of depression, a lingering feeling of intense sadness that can interfere with daily life by keeping you from going to work or school or caring for your children. Studies show that depression can increase your risk of developing CVD or of dying from the condition if you already have CVD. In fact, depression and social isolation are powerful psychosocial risk factors for CVD, both for the initial development and progress toward recurrent heart attacks.

Exactly how depression increases the risk of heart disease is not known. But we do know that depression is surprisingly common.

In a recent study I conducted, nearly 40 percent of women in our hospital recovering from a heart attack or bypass surgery had clinical depression. Many times, it goes undetected because physicians don't ask about it. I've noticed that many male patients are especially uncomfortable talking about depression. I had one high-level executive in my care who had undergone bypass surgery, was diagnosed with diabetes and lost his father before he finally opened up to the idea he might be depressed and agreed to treatment. And even then, it was a struggle.

One concern we have about patients with depression is they may be less apt to take their medication as directed. There's an identifiable link between being depressed and not being compliant with medical recommendations and eventually ending up in the hospital. Depression may also enhance the physiological pathways by which CVD develops. One study showed, for example, that depression might increase levels of C-reactive protein, an inflammatory marker that has been associated with increased risk of heart attack. It's a murky area in medicine, but one thing is clear: depression often goes under the radar because nearly two-thirds of those with depression don't seek treatment.

We all have times when we don't feel up to snuff. But depression is more than "the blues." It's an illness that requires individual or group psychotherapy and/or antidepressant medication to treat it. According to the National Institutes of Mental Health, such treatment is effective in 80 percent of all cases. Because depression can cloud thinking, those with depression can't always help themselves. Suspect you may be suffering from depression? See your doctor, who can conduct a quick and easy screening test to determine if you need a referral and/or treatment. Here's a tool that was used in the INTERHEART study I mentioned earlier. If you answer yes to the first question and then yes to any five out of seven of the others, you may have clinical depression and should seek help from a physician.

Depression Screening Test

Please answer yes or no to the following questions:

1. During the past twelve months, was there ever a time when you felt sad, blue or depressed for two weeks or more in a row?
2. If yes, during those times, did you:
   — Lose interest in most things like hobbies, work or activities that usually give you pleasure?
   — Feel tired or low on energy?
   — Gain or lose weight?
   — Have more trouble falling asleep than you usually do?
   — Have more trouble concentrating than usual?
   — Think a lot about death (either your own, someone else's or death in general)?
   —Feel down on yourself, no good or worthless?

Getting Over Getting Dumped (By My Bike)

I sought help for depression by making an appointment with my gynecologist after I had been in a bicycle crash when I was training for a triathlon with my husband. I had hit a crevice in the pavement and went flying over the handlebars, which injured my shoulder. I was lucky, because my smashed shoulder could have been much worse. Still, I was in for a summer of physical therapy and out of my element because I wasn't able to exercise. Plus, I had to cancel all of my triathlons. It was a major downer. I knew I wasn't taking it well and needed some help.

"I think I'm depressed," I told my gynecologist. "I cry easily. I'm sad. I'm upset and short with my kids. I think it's temporary and related to my bike accident, but maybe I need treatment." My self-diagnosis made it easy for her to just write me out a prescription, but she wasn't buying it.

"Lori, you don't need a drug," she said gently. "You just need to get physically active again." Initially, I was mad. Then I realized that maybe she was right. So as soon as I got home, I started walking like crazy (that's one thing I could still do), and within a few weeks, I was my old self again. I needed to focus on what I could do instead of what I couldn't do.

That was a good lesson. There are lots of different antidepressants available these days to help alleviate depression, but as with CVD, lifestyle therapy may be an important remedy.

What To Do When Someone You Love Is Depressed

If you suspect a friend or family member may be suffering from depression, here's what you can do to ease their suffering and help keep his or her heart healthy.

Take quick action. Symptoms of depression include persistent sadness or irritability, being unable to concentrate, withdrawal, difficulty falling and staying asleep, sleeping much less or more than usual, poor appetite, weight loss, slowed speech, and/or intense feelings of guilt. In extreme cases, those suffering from depression may talk about ending their lives, hurting themselves or others, or giving away all of their possessions. According to the NIMH, about 15 percent of people with depression experience this kind of suicidal behavior. If you know someone who fits this description, get involved.

It's not normal for people to be talking about the end of their lives. For starters, approach that person and say, "You seem abnormally depressed. You're talking about ending your life. I think it's time to get help." Contacting emergency medical services or your state's local office of mental health (check your phone book) is an option when the situation seems urgent. There may be a mobile crisis unit that disperses a team of mental health professionals to evaluate the person in danger. You may feel funny working behind a loved one's back to get him into treatment, but you don't want to be looking back saying, "Gee, I wish I had done something."

Get involved. If you know someone showing nonsuicidal signs of depression, such as persistent sadness or irritability, withdrawal, and/or weight loss, again, don't ignore it. Out of concern, approach that person, but tread lightly. You might say, "You look different. Is there something wrong?" If your friend or loved one says nothing's wrong, you might say, "Are you sure?" Then get specific. For example, you might say, "I've noticed you're not yourself at work lately. You seem depressed. I'm concerned, and I want to help." If your loved one is receptive to what you're saying, hear him or her out. Then, as a starting point, suggest they call their family doctor, who may be trained to treat a certain range of mental health conditions. Or recommend someone else to see. You might also offer to go with them to the doctor or therapist appointment. Feel like you're interfering? Don't. Getting involved like this can strengthen the bond you have with people who are depressed and help you, too.

Too Blessed to Be Stressed: The Art of Saying Thank You

In my experience, my patients who are grateful for what they have, instead of anxious about what they don't, also do the very best. I believe the degree to which we're thankful just for being alive is predictive of heart health. This isn't documented in scientific research, but I think it's physiologically impossible to be thankful and stressed at the same time. So I often encourage my patients, when they're particularly burdened, to take a few deep breaths and think about what they are thankful for. Try it for yourself the next time your life is at the boiling point.

I'm also a believer in the healing power of writing actual thank-you notes. In fact, I consider writing thank-you notes a life skill that's important for heart health. To this day, when I write a thank-you note, I feel good. I might even shed a few tears. There's so much human kindness we don't acknowledge. But when we do, we feel less stress and anger toward the world because, through the written act of thanking someone, we internalize our gratefulness, and our hearts benefit. To me, writing thank-you notes is an opportunity to heal myself, not a sacrifice of time.

My sentiments stem from—who else—good ol' Mom. For every Christmas or birthday present I received as a child, my mother made me write a thank-you note. Although I often resented writing those letters as a child, the habit has served me well in adulthood. Sometimes when I feel overwhelmed, I write a thank-you to someone to whom I owe appreciation, to remind myself just how lucky I really am. And now I'm carrying on the tradition with my own kids. They may feel annoyed to take the time to write a thank-you note to someone, for example, for coming to their birthday party, but it helps them realize that their friends cared enough about them to come, which builds self-esteem, and that's clearly important for health and well-being.

Quick, Grab a Pen!

I can't tell you how wonderful it feels to read the thank-you notes my husband, who is a pediatric cardiac surgeon, gets from the grateful parents of the children he has operated on. Many of these children had hearts that were almost beyond repair—no fault of their own or anyone else's. But now they have a chance to live and love. Considering the complexity of the heart, having a healthy one truly is a miracle. If I could, I would write God a thank-you note for my own healthy heart. I would!

To whom do you owe a debt of gratitude? Do you have a word of thanks that's long overdue to someone who did you a favor or performed an unrequited act of human kindness for no other reason than just to be nice? Go ahead and heal your heart and write your thank-you note here. You don't have to send it, but I think you should.

_____

_____

_____

_____

_____

_____

_____

A Love Letter to Syracuse, Where All Things Are Possible

Need inspiration? Here's an excerpt from actual thank-you note I recently wrote to the City of Syracuse, which was published in the local newspaper, the *Post Standard.* I wrote it after I learned that I was going to receive the Outstanding Young Alumni award from Upstate Medical University. Of course, the best way to say thank-you in life is to do a good job and enjoy what you do. But I think it's important to literally express it whenever possible because it is reinforcing to those you are thanking—and then maybe they will thank someone else. At the risk of sounding trite, I think that if we all just focused a little more on our thank-you notes, the world would be a much better place.

To the City of Syracuse:

All that I have been able to experience and accomplish is a testimony to this unique, wonderful city that progressively embraced the idea that everyone, regardless of their social and economic status, deserves a chance.

I was fortunate to be one of the test cases for a City of Syracuse recreational program targeted to low- and middle-income kids that allowed me to swim competitively year-round, kept me out of trouble, and provided access to Syracuse University facilities and coaches. I didn't know then that the discipline and perseverance I learned as a Syracuse Charger would be invaluable to me later in life as a physician-scientist. Moreover, I have been able to share the healthful life skills I learned with my own children.

I didn't know how lucky I was at Henninger High School when the athletic director tolerated me swimming on the boys' team. Before Title IX there was no equivalent for girls. That experience would help prepare me to work alongside my colleagues in cardiovascular medicine, when I was frequently the only female on the team.

When my high school raised money to send me on an American Field Service International exchange program to Sweden, I didn't know that one day I would chair the first International Conference on Women and Heart Disease to bring leaders and the medical profession together to combat a burgeoning global epidemic. My exchange experience made the world seem smaller and underscored how each person can make a difference.

To this day, it still baffles my mother that it took me so long and so many advanced degrees to understand and teach the public what she instilled in me as a child, to "eat your fruits and vegetables, and get exercise every day."

I have learned the magnitude of her wisdom and a lot of other things in my studies and travels over the past twenty years. But if there is one thing that I have always known, it is that there really is no place like Syracuse and no place I'm prouder to call home.

Getting Off the Treadmill

I particularly recall a thank-you note I wrote to my son's kindergarten teacher in Michigan, three years after my youngest son Mike was in her class. We didn't even live in the same state anymore. But hey, it's never too late to give thanks where it's due, is it? The background of the story is that two weeks into the school year, I got a call from Mike's teacher. Mike was a five-year-old with a lot of energy; let's use the word "spirited." That much I knew, and that never bothered me, because frankly, I'm kind of spirited, too. But put Mike in a group of thirty kids, and spirited becomes disruptive, the teacher informed me. "Mike is really smart," she said, "but he's going to have trouble if he doesn't play by the rules. He's got to learn to not talk so much and to be calmer."

There are lots of ways you can handle that kind of situation. Initially I got defensive. *There's something wrong with this school,* I thought. *Here I've got a high-energy, smart kid, and the school just wants to squelch his individuality.* I briskly thanked her and hung up the phone!

Over the next weeks and months, however, her words began to sink in. I began to recognize a pattern. When we'd go on vacation and be together as a family for a week, we noticed that Mike would be calmer. Conversely, when I'd travel, Mike would really start to act out in school.

Admittedly, at that point in my life, I was constantly being pulled in a dozen directions and flying to research meetings as part of my full-time job as director of Preventive Cardiology at the University of Michigan. To be successful in research and medicine, it is necessary to travel to multicenter clinical meetings and advisory boards, as well as participate in government task forces. Each one of those is an opportunity that helps fuel a medical career. There are certain milestones you have to hit at designated times, or those chances for advancement are often gone forever.

Meanwhile, I was also working on my Ph.D., and my husband, Ralph, was starting his career in pediatric cardiac surgery. Needless to say, it was a stressful time in our lives. It seemed as though there was no getting off the treadmill.

To bridge the gaps, we hired au pairs, and everything seemed to be working out well. I was so proud of myself for doing a good job juggling work and family. Or so I thought, until I began putting the pieces of the puzzle together. Mike's behavior was probably fueled by anxiety, I finally surmised, after a few more meetings with his teacher. He never knew when I'd be traveling next. The au pair was fine, but she just wasn't me.

We all like to think we're spending enough time with our kids, but over the next few months, I began to recognize my own denial. It became clear to me that the decisions I was making to further my career were having a negative impact on my family, especially my rambunctious kindergartener. Some adjustments were in order. Initially, I began taking Mike to the school bus stop, relieving the au pair of that responsibility. I realized that getting on the bus is an apprehensive time for children, and it was better if I was there. Then I nixed the idea of an au pair altogether, cut way back on my travel, and concentrated on spending more time with Mike and my other son, Matt. Just hanging out and helping with homework and other projects, being there for them, became more the norm.

Believe me, it is so much easier to write about that period of my life than it was to live it. It killed me to have to start declining professional opportunities that arose. What was I afraid of? If I began saying no to this and that, I was afraid no one would want me to serve on important committees. I was convinced it was the end of my career. On a practical level, it was tough, too. Hands down, going to work was a lot easier than raising inquisitive, energetic children.

Still, the changes I made proved to be win/win in the long run. When I began saying no, I had more time to concentrate on the really important aspects of my work, which made me more enduring in the long run. And by the end of the school year, there was an amazing difference in Mike. He was calm, confident—like a different kid. It

؛ an enormous payoff. But without that teacher's insight and constant encouragement, I would have never dealt with it or seen it. She helped me so much with that aspect of childrearing. It would have been easier for the teacher to avoid confronting me, especially about that issue—how much time I'm spending with my kid—which is a touchy subject for many parents.

So I wrote her a note to let her know how wonderfully Mike was doing in the later years of elementary school and to thank her for her insight. Had I not made those adjustments and reduced my schedule, I am not sure how well Mike would have done. Thanking her in writing reinforced the importance of making that difficult life decision, and to feel the rewards that came with facing them. Learning these important lessons is instrumental in prevention, too. Cutting out excess to focus on the important things in life is healing.

Overcoming Mommy Guilt

If you're a working mom, you probably know what I mean when I say that the guilt factor can be strong. No matter how you readjust your work schedule to spend more time with your kids, you feel as though you should be investing more time with them, and more, and more. And as I mentioned in my thank-you letter to Mike's kindergarten teacher, sometimes you actually do need to put in more time on the home front. But sometimes you don't have to. In fact, when Mike was nine and Matt was twelve, I again went through a long period of asking myself, "Am I doing the right thing by spending the time I do on my career? Is it negatively impacting my children—in ways I just can't see?"

I needed help with this issue, so one day, when Mike was getting dressed for school, I went into his room. "Mike, can I talk to you for a minute?" I asked. "I've got a problem, and I need your help." I told Mike that I was thinking of not working anymore. "I'm worried that I'm not spending enough time with you and Matt," I confessed. "Should I just stop working?" I asked him.

With a puzzled, "what-are-you-crazy?" look on his face, Mike said, "Mom, we see plenty of you. And besides, you love your job, and you help people eat better." Mike's response was a turning point for me. I realized that my guilt was coming from me, not my kids. I was giving them enough of me. They were fine, and in fact, I couldn't have taught them the lesson they learned by watching me if I stayed home and said to them every day, "Find a meaningful job you love, and be happy." But remember, we don't have to be all things to all people at all times. I had paid my dues with my kids by spending time with them when they really needed it when they were little. I had built the foundation. Now I could do both. And giving up the guilt contributes to a destressed and heart-healthy life.

Personalizing Your Destress Routine

Carving out personal time, dealing with depression, building up a support system and writing thank-you notes are just a few of the things I do, and suggest you do, too, to heal our hearts and counteract the stresses of daily life. But there may be other things that might work for you. In fact, like having brown eyes and curly hair or looking better in blue than in chartreuse, relaxation is very individual. According to stress experts, there are four basic stress "types," which are based on our personalities and temperaments. The four stress types are: Monitors, Distracters, Spiritually Inclined and Fidgeters. (Some of us may be a mix of more than one stress type.) What's your stress type? Read on to find out. When you become aware of your stress type, you can fine-tune your personal stress-reduction program to highlight your strengths and increase your comfort level.

Type 1: The Monitor

The Monitor's modus operendom is control. You like to live in the present at all times and ask a lot of questions during stressful situations. Despite having an active imagination, you find it nearly impossible to find time to calm down and mentally get away from the source of stress. The Monitor's mind can be his/her worst enemy when it comes to relaxing and finding their center of peace. You know you're a Monitor if:

- In the doctor or the dentist office, for example, you keep your eyes open and stay focused on what's going on around you. You tend to inquire about every little poke and prod. ("Um . . . now what are you doing?")
- Asked to imagine yourself, say, walking through a peaceful forest, you either get a blank screen or can't focus on the image for more than a few seconds.
- You tend to focus on the *what ifs* when you're under stress. What if you get in a car accident over the weekend and miss your Monday deadline? What if you trip when you're walking down the aisle at your best friend's wedding? What if one of your kids gets sick, but you can't miss any more days at work?

Stress Rx for Monitors: If you think you're a Monitor, here's a program you can institute daily or when you think you need to: breathe, breathe. A couple of conscious breaths work wonders, especially for this stress type. No matter where you are, simply sit upright and bring your awareness to your breathing. Follow your breath as it goes in and comes out of your body. Feel your belly fill with breath. You might even want to place your hand on your abdomen and feel it rise and fall in sync with each breath.

Type 2: The Distracter

If you're a Distracter, you would rather stick your head in the sand during stressful situations and not know the details. You find it easy to mentally escape, and you want to. You know you're a Distracter if:

- During a medical procedure, you maintain a let-me-know-when-it's-over mind-set. You're inclined to say, "Just give me the big picture," or, "Don't tell me."
- During a choppy airplane ride, you find it easy to sleep or escape into a good book. You also want to be spared the pilot's play-by-play on the PA system.
- In general, you find it relatively easy to mentally escape. When your boss drops yet another project on your desk, you take a quick, mental time-out and imagine yourself, say, sipping margaritas on the veranda at sunset. Ahh . . .

Stress Rx for Distracters: If this sounds like you, use your gift for mentally escaping by using your talents for creative visualization. Imagine yourself somewhere better during trying times—but don't focus on just any mental image. Try different scenarios and pick one *you* truly find relaxing. Keep engaging reading material and your favorite videos on hand for instant escapism.

You might also try this variation on meditation: focus on an interesting object in the room or a complex and meaningful thought, something that gets your mind involved. Also, turn to music. Concentrate on the instruments, or remember a time or a place associated with the song or artist. For stress relief on the run, tote a Walkman or a handheld CD player stocked with tunes that soothe you. Also, arm yourself with engaging reading materials, such as a good book or magazine. At home, stock your video library with your preferred picks.

Type 3: The Spiritually Inclined

You're spiritually inclined if you especially feel a reverent connection to the universe. Whether or not you participate in any organized religion, you believe there is a higher power that gives you direction in your life and protects you. You know you're Spiritually Inclined if:

- Repeating a prayer or a spiritual mantra or word that signifies peace during anxious times has a calming, comforting impact on you.
- You feel a deep sacredness of all things, like the splendor of a spring day or the divinity of a sunset.

Stress Rx for the Spiritually Inclined: Repeating a short, spiritual concentration phrase, such as, "God is with me," is probably your best antidote for stressful moments. (Secular mantras such as, "Be calm," or, "Cool, relaxed mind, calm body," may do nothing for you.) Again, choose a spiritual phrase that resonates with you.

Connect with nature. For general stress relief, embrace nature. Get into the habit of going for a leisurely walk in the park, sitting by a river or the ocean, or watching the sunset or birds at a bird feeder.

If you don't already, try attending religious services every so often. You may be comforted by the hymns or simply the feeling of connection with others.

Type 4: The Fidgeter

The Fidgeter needs to do some form of exercise to find even marginal stress relief. Physically passive relaxation techniques, such as using a mantra sans movement or meditation—focusing on a neutral object, such as a candle flame, and clearing your head from daily chatter—often don't work. You know you're a Fidgeter if:

RED-HOT

RED-CARPET STYLE

Best Deal

CHECK ONE:

☐ 24 monthly issues for just $1.49 per issue.   ☐ 12 monthly issues for just $1.69 per issue.

Plus 30¢ per issue postage and handling

ONLY $1.49 an issue

Name (please print)

Address   Apt. No.

City   State   Zip

E-mail

☐ Payment enclosed.   ☐ Bill me later.

INAPWS4

08IINIBJ

For faster service, call 1-800-633-6355 or visit instyle.com/order

InStyle

- You've got energy to burn; just the thought of sitting still through even a manicure or a pedicure, for example, is enough to drive you batty.
- You feel destressed after exercise—even though during your workout, your mind may wander to the memo you didn't write, your outfit for dinner with your potential in-laws, whether your baby is due for a checkup.
- You're a master at multitasking—and think nothing of say, putting on your makeup during the morning while talking on your phone, sipping coffee and spewing out directions to the kids.

Stress Rx for Fidgeters: In general, fidgeters need techniques that engage body and mind to achieve a deep sense of mental and physical relaxation. Your best bet: take part in a walking (moving) meditation. That is, while walking, concentrate on feeling your feet touch the ground with each step while silently repeating a soothing phrase such as, "Easy does it." This exercise helps you focus your mind in the present moment. Otherwise, you're apt to walk and worry and deprive yourself of that much-needed mental break. Exercise in general is also beneficial, but it's important to choose an activity that demands your undivided attention. Team sports, dance classes or terrain-challenging mountain biking also work well.

Three Keys to Your Heart

Here are three key points I hope you'll take to heart. Consider them my take-away tasks from this chapter.

1. **Don't discount your mental health.** It may be just as important a risk factor for CVD as physiological factors such as blood pressure and cholesterol. Try downsizing stress. Take time out for yourself daily, write thank-you notes and allow yourself a good soak in the tub. If these don't work for you, find something that does. Stress reduction is individual, but you may need to work at it. In our to-do-driven society, it doesn't always come easily.

2. **If you think you or a loved one is depressed, follow up with a doctor or other mental health professional.** Don't think it will just go away by itself. You can't will depression away, although certain lifestyle changes, like exercise, can help keep it at bay. Still, you may be a candidate for treatment. Depression is a significant risk factor for CVD.

3. **Give your children opportunities to destress, too.** Teaching them how to calm down and center themselves is a life skill that can serve them well now and into adulthood and to help keep their hearts healthy. It's an aspect we often overlook, but it's just as important as formal education and SAT scores.

Chapter

5

Exercising for the Health of It

"There is a choice you have to make in everything you do. You must always keep in mind the choice you make makes you."

—Anonymous

I'll never forget the day it came time to take the swimming test to pass the beginner's swimming class. It feels like yesterday. I was seven years old, and all I had to do was put my head under water, float and kick. At that point, I hadn't actually floated yet, but I really wanted to pass so I could stay in the pool without a parent, which was the rule at our neighborhood pool. One by one, each kid was asked to push off the wall and kick a short distance with arms outstretched, face in the water. When my turn finally came, I could barely contain my excitement. I pushed off the wall and floated for the first time. Yeah! I did it!

Or so I thought. I was more like a missile headed straight to the bottom. After the class, the teacher sat us down on benches in the locker room for what turned out to be a defining moment in my life. Down the line, she said, "You pass," to each swimmer. But when she came to me, the last, she paused. I was so nervous; I swore my heart was beating out of my chest. "You need to be a little stronger swimmer before I can pass you," she said. My heart sank with sadness and humiliation. How could I have failed a beginning swimming class? No kid likes to hear she's not good at something or to fail in front of her friends. There is a lot of pressure for kids to be good at sports, and experiences like this can discourage kids. Sports are supposed to be fun; they're to be played, not graded. But after I got over my initial devastation, I literally dove right back in, with my father, who loved to swim, as my teacher.

Dad didn't have a lot of spare time. In the summer months, he'd work from 6 A.M. until 3 P.M. as a mail carrier. At 5 P.M., he'd head to a second job. Still, he had a two-hour window every day. You'd think he'd take a nap or watch TV. Not my dad. "Come on kids, let's go swimming," he'd say. And we'd all suit up and head down to the neighborhood pool.

Although I was learning swimming skills, it was unbeknownst to me because swimming became a game and playtime with my family and friends. It was more fun than anything else. "There are numbers on the drain, and anybody who comes up with those numbers gets seven cents for a Fudgsicle," Dad would say. We'd dive again and again, never, of course, getting the numbers quite right because there actually weren't any on the drain. It was just Dad's way of teaching and motivating us to learn to swim. Over the course of that summer, and after a few dozen Fudgsicles just for the effort, I apparently got pretty good at swimming, because the next year, the very same lifeguard who failed me asked me to be on the swim team. It's true—success *is* the best revenge!

"You've got to call your father," my mother said when I won my first blue ribbon in a swim meet. So I rang him at the post office, crying with joy. It must have taken me five minutes to explain that no, I hadn't hurt myself. I had won the twenty-five-yard freestyle for the eight-year-olds and under! I still have that faded blue ribbon.

Long story short, I was hooked. From there, I began to swim year-round as a member of a competitive swim team called the Syracuse Chargers, a swimming program targeted to low- to middle-income kids that didn't charge any fees. Numerous competitions and the Junior Olympics followed, consuming my summers. In high school, I wanted to keep swimming, but in those pre–Title IX times in the 1970s, a girls' swim team simply didn't exist. "Well, I'll just swim on the boys' team then," I said, which was met with resistance. "Where will you change if the visiting team uses the girls' locker room?" I was asked. "I'll use the janitor's closet next to the pool," I responded. There was a will, and there was a way, and the powers that be could see that. I was allowed to swim, and that's all I cared about. After I broke several school records for the boys, the school started a girls' swim team the following year, and we went on to be league champions, a victory for all of us. I won the fifty-yard butterfly at the sectional championships. I can still hear the cheers of my female teammates because they knew I had won before I did.

In college and throughout medical school, I continued to swim competitively. Even though I was on call every other or every third night, I swam every chance I got. I also worked as a lifeguard at the medical school pool, which is where I met my husband (now married twenty years!), who was also a competitive swimmer and a former captain of his college team at Davidson, North Carolina. Swimming became my life skill for stress relief and, indeed, it served me well. There were many advantages to this lifelong sport!

In the early 1980s, just as I was graduating from medical school, triathlons started to become popular. Hmm, I thought. I could swim. I was a decent runner. All I needed to do was learn how to ride a bicycle with gears. (I hadn't had one growing up because we just didn't have money for such a bicycle.) But with the monetary gifts I received at my graduation, which added up to $1,000—a million dollars to me at the time—I bought a $999 silver triathlon bicycle I had my eye on the very next day. Two weeks later, after my husband taught me how to shift gears, I competed in my first triathlon and came in second overall. One thing led to another, and before I knew it, I qualified to compete in the ultimate triathlon, the Hawaii Ironman. Fortunately, my colleagues at Syracuse Veterans Administration Hospital, where I was working at the time, were supportive, granting me time to train and compete. All in all, it was a great race—12 hours, 22 minutes and 27 seconds. I finished twenty-sixth in the world in my division, after swimming 2.4 miles, cycling for 112 miles and running a 26.2-mile marathon. Whew! And to think it all started with just having fun and diving for numbers with Dad at the local swimming pool.

There are so many more levels to participating in endurance sports than just the exercise components. It is such an enriching experience to become one with nature while participating in activities such as I have described. I have felt on occasion that it is a truly religious experience. I never feel more connected to God than when I'm running along with my heart pounding, the wind in my hair and the blinding sun on my face.

Finishing the Ironman was a life-changing event for me. It was close to midnight on October 22, 1988, when my husband drove me back to our hotel. I could barely move without cramping up, so he gently tucked me into bed. I took his hand and thanked him for being patient and being there for me. I looked him in the eyes and said, "I'm done now. I did what I needed to do. Let's start our family next year." The next morning, I bought a souvenir "Iron Baby" mesh T-shirt, size 3 to 6 months. As irony and the gods would have it, our son Matthew, which means "gift of God," was born on

October 22, 1989, exactly a year later. I joked with my husband through the long, torturous labor that it was a lot like the Ironman. The contractions would come in waves and remind me of the ups and downs of the ocean swells and the ascents and descents on the long bike ride. My long hours of active labor were a lot like the painful marathon on the Queen K. The big difference was that at least on the marathon I knew where the turnaround was!

It turns out there was more irony to that Iron Baby T-shirt than delivering a baby on the one-year anniversary of completing the Hawaii Ironman. Matthew, my Iron Baby, turned out to be quite the triathlete. Last summer, he and I started racing in sprint triathlons together, and in October 1994, he won the U.S. National Sprint Triathlon Championships for males ages fourteen and under, in Lake Charles, Louisiana. He is now competing and training all over North America. One day, he hopes to make the Olympic trials. But he has a much more formidable goal than that—to someday complete the Hawaii Ironman with his mom!

Sports can be a special bond you share with your whole family. Ralph, Matt and I love to train and race together, although we have a hard time keeping up with Matt now. Our second son, Mike, is a diver and gymnast, which seems to run in the family as I also competed in gymnastics for many years. We love to train on the trampoline together. Instead of diving for numbers and Fudgsicles like my dad challenged me to do, we jump and do goofy stunts for the prize of who doesn't have to do the dishes!

Still the Only Girl on the Boys' Team

I learned so much from those early experiences in sports, skills that have carried me through life. As a specialist in preventive cardiology, I'm often one of the few women, and sometimes the only woman, on the professional boards I'm on, because cardio-vascular medicine is comprised mostly of men. But I've learned that when you have a shared mission—whether it's swimming to win or preventing heart disease—gender issues melt away. Nobody cares whether you're a man or a woman when you have the common ground of a collective passion. What really matters is getting the job done.

The discipline I gained from training and competing in athletics has also been invaluable to me as a researcher. Success in academic preventive cardiology is challenging and requires lots of patience and endurance, like pouring the last drop from the honey jar. There are many failures before success, and the persistence it takes can be daunting. Scientific papers and grants need to be constantly revised after the peer review process. It takes a thick skin and determination to respond to criticism. But if you can tough it out, the process works, and the final product is something you can be proud of.

I remember when I chaired the expert panel and wrote the evidenced-based guidelines for CVD prevention in women, a landmark paper that was a monumental task and needed to be completed in less than a year. The panel had to review a system-atic search of several thousand scientific research studies to find the best science to make clinical recommendations. We then had to bring twelve major professional and government organizations to consensus and get another twenty-two organizations to approve and endorse the wording of almost thirty recommendations and the quality of the evidence to support each of them. I had to lead a series of teleconferences of experts from many different back-grounds and perspectives and bring them together. Votes were tal-lied, recommendations were revised and sent to dozens of reviewers, then rewritten again. Words like "consistently" and "regularly" were debated. Commas and semicolons received meticulous attention to prevent any misunderstandings.

As I was nearing the end, just as at the Hawaii Ironman years before, I had to muster the energy to complete the task on time. I had a flashback of the conclusion of the race and crossing the finish line (nearly crawling, I might add). That's when I found the inner strength to clear the finish line in my professional life and complete the mission because I had been able to do it before in my athletic life. Exercise and sports build a wealth of inner resources we can draw upon for many things in life.

When you're faced with a challenge in your personal or professional life and need to rise to the occasion, I encourage you to think of a physical feat you've accomplished but didn't think you could, or even create one by setting new fitness goals. Your physical strength and endurance can set a precedent for enduring the mental and emotional rigors of daily life. It's the "if I can do that, then I can do this" school of thought that facilitates this type of accomplishment.

Exercise Rx

Just like any other muscle, the heart (also a muscle) gets stronger with exercise. But besides increasing your physical strength and stamina, physical activity also lowers blood pressure, raises HDL (the "good") cholesterol, lowers triglycerides, dilates blood vessels to improve circulation and provides an anti-inflammatory response, all of which benefits heart health.

To this day, I still compete in triathlons, but for the fitness benefits and pleasure of it, rather than the competition. (I get plenty of that in my professional life!) But don't worry. To live a heart-healthy life, you don't have to be a triathlete. You don't even have to exercise long or intensely. When I convey to my patients how important exercise is for heart health, they don't ask me how much exercise they need to prevent heart disease. They ask, "How little do I need to do?" My response is always met with relief, "You don't have to do very much." For heart health, investing just thirty minutes of moderately intense physical activity, such as brisk walking, swimming, cycling, dancing, gardening and/or yard work most days of the week is all you need to do your heart good. That's all you need to do, but it's vital.

In fact, I recently told a patient who needed to improve his cholesterol profile, "This is the most important prescription a doctor is ever going to give you. It's the perfect medicine." I jotted on my pad, "Exercise thirty minutes/day" and handed the paper to him. Then I got even more specific and told him to go walking for thirty minutes with his family every night at the neighborhood track, which he told me was just minutes from his house, instead of watching TV after dinner. "Walking at the track is going to help prevent your kids from becoming obese." (He told me they were on the heavy side.) "It's going to help keep your wife from developing high blood pressure and high cholesterol, and it's going to treat yours." And to drive my point home, I summarized, "It will also provide the added benefit of giving you more quality family time," which I sensed they really needed. We have a motto in our house: "The family that plays together, stays together." I share this with my patients to encourage them to exercise together, too.

The bottom line is that exercise not only makes you look and feel better, it improves your overall well-being. There isn't a pharmaceutical known to man that does all the good things that exercise does, and it has almost no negative side effects, especially if you do low-impact activities, such as brisk walking. And you can even break up that thirty minutes per day into three ten-minute bouts of, for example, ten minutes of brisk walking on your way to work, ten minutes on your lunch hour and ten minutes on your way home. Your heart doesn't care when you do it, just how much you do.

One of the easiest ways to help you reach that daily thirty-minute goal is to wear a step counter (pedometer) and work toward accumulating at least 10,000 steps per day. A pedometer gives you credit for all the physical activity you may have been doing all along, but weren't necessarily counting as "exercise," such as gardening, walking the dog daily, trekking to and from your car at work, playing with your kids at the playground, or hauling the laundry basket up and down the stairs several times a week. Those sorts of lifestyle behaviors aren't as rigorous or as structured as a gym workout, but they can make a difference and convey heart-health benefits.

"Exercise thirty minutes/day"

Go ahead and write this prescription on a piece of paper and put it in a place where you'll see it often, such as on your refrigerator or the dashboard of your car, as a reminder.

Your Walking Workout— A Step in the Right Direction

If you're not used to daily walking, then walk slowly and take short, frequent walks, gradually increasing distance and speed. Start slowly, with five to ten minutes of walking, and gradually working your way up to thirty minutes. The key is to just get started and keep at it. Getting back to or into the fitness game is all about setting a small goal, meeting it, feeling good about it and then setting a new goal that's a little bit harder.

In fact, once you've mastered doing thirty minutes of moderately intense activity, you may want to up the ante if you also want to shed pounds, prevent weight gain or get fit (not just reap heart-health benefits). To walk for weight management, for example, you'll need to walk sixty minutes a day at least four days a week according to the current USDA recommendations for physical activity. If your goal is to get aerobically fit, the American College of Sports Medicine recommends walking faster—to the point at which you're winded or at 60 percent of your maximum heart rate (a good approximation is 220 minus your age; for example, if you're forty years old, 220–40 = 180) at least three times a week for at least twenty minutes.

Ideally, to get all three benefits and avoid boredom, it's good to mix and match. On days you have less time, you can walk faster, but for twenty to thirty minutes. On others, like the weekend, you can walk for an hour or even longer, but more leisurely. And for days when you're really busy, you work in thirty minutes of walking here and there during the course of your day.

With these basic guidelines in mind, the following are effective ways to help you reach your goals, whether you're walking for heart health, to manage weight or get fit—or a combination of all three.

Pay attention to your pace. No matter what your goals, knowing how fast you're walking is important. For basic health benefits, a "health pace" of 120 steps per minute (3 miles per hour) is what you're after. For weight loss, aim for 135 steps per minute (4 miles per hour), and for fitness, 145 to 150 steps per minute (4.5 miles per hour) should be your goal. To quickly estimate, simply count your steps for twenty seconds as you walk, then multiply by three for a per-minute step rate. Are you walking too slowly or too fast for your goal? Now you'll know. Depending on your goals, the key steps to hit at the 20-second mark are 40, 45 or 50.

Fix your form. For maximum efficiency, make sure you're walking with proper form. To do that, concentrate on standing tall, keeping your shoulders back and focusing on the horizon as you walk rather than looking down or at your feet. If you want to gain speed, you'll want to take quicker steps, not longer ones, and bend your arms. As you swing your arms, your hands should trace an arc from your waistband to your chest. An exaggerated swing—swinging your arms up to your chin and your elbows back behind you, like the caricature of a race walker—will slow you down. The best arm swing is natural, close and compact. Faster arms will make your feet move faster. Finally, for greater momentum and power, push off with your toes at the end of every step. You should feel as if you're shoving the sole of your shoe into someone behind you.

Don't weight your gait. Wearing wrist, ankle and waist weights, as well as a weighted vest, while you walk may burn more calories, but it also changes your gait, putting strain on joints and can possibly lead to injury, especially considering that you do thousands of reps when you walk. If you want the benefits of both weight training and walking, it's safer to do them separately. If you want to build muscle, take an extra ten minutes after your walk and lift ten- to fifteen-pound weights rather than really light ones.

A more effective way to burn more calories aerobically, and add variety to your walking workout, is to include a hilly route in your repertoire or raise the incline periodically on the treadmill, and keep your step-rate pace up as you climb. If you slow down to compensate for the incline, you won't gain much benefit.

You can also go off-road. You expend more calories if you walk on rougher surfaces, such as trails compared to sidewalks or a track, because you'll use smaller leg muscles that help maintain balance. It's a different kind of intensity.

Keep an activity log. Noting your daily activity is a great motivator, especially when you see those miles or steps (if you have a pedometer) start to build up. Shoot for 10,000 steps a day for health; 12,000 to 15,000 steps per day for weight loss; and for aerobic fitness, make sure 3,000 to 6,000 steps are at an increased speed. Tally your daily, weekly and monthly totals.

Another motivational trick is to be proactive and prioritize walking or another activity by scheduling it in your day planner and setting external rewards. You might, for example, put $5 in an envelope each week you meet your exercise objectives. At the end of the month you can buy yourself something nice. Just be sure that you only reward yourself if you meet your goal.

Also, keep your athletic shoes somewhere you're going to see them, whether it's in your car or by the front door, so you're always ready to go. It's important to have a visual reminder that exercise is a priority.

A NOTE FROM DR. LORI: BABY STEPS

If there is ever a day when you're just too tired to go for a walk, don't talk yourself out of it. Those days always turn out to be the best ones. To stay on track, I play a game with myself. I say, "I'm too tired to do this today, so I will just do a block." Then I get out there and say, "Okay, just one more," and before I know it, I've done three miles and feel like a new, energized, stress-relieved person! The key is to avoid setting expectations that are too high. It's always better to start with baby steps and build from there.

Fitting In Exercise

For all of us, exercising just thirty minutes each day is doable. Still, too few of us do it. According to the U.S. Surgeon General, more than 60 percent of Americans don't get enough physical activity, and more than 25 percent of us aren't active at all. Over the years, I've heard many excuses from my patients regarding why they don't exercise: "I don't like to sweat. It will mess up my hair. I'm too tired, too old, too busy. The weather's bad. I'm embarrassed because everyone at the gym is already thin." Perhaps the most common excuse I hear is, "I don't have time." To that, I always ask, "Do you not have time to exercise, or are you simply not expending the time?"

Of course, we're all busy, but I suspect for most of us we choose not to expend the time we have on exercise. The time does exist. In fact, I know it does. To prove my point—that everyone has thirty minutes each day to exercise—I just look at the math in the following chart, which shows where our time goes in a given week, for an average person. Take a look.

SOLUTION FOR THE "NO TIME TO EXERCISE" EXCUSE

Total hours per week	168
Sleep 8 hours per night	- 56
Work 9 hours/day x 5 days	- 45
Travel 1 hour to/from work	- 10
Cleaning/Grooming 1 hour/day	- 7
Errands 1.5 hours/day	- 10.5
Family time 1.5 hours/day	- 10.5
Social/religious activities	- 10
Miscellaneous (such as cooking) 1 hour/day	- 7

Total = 156
(leaves 12 hours to "make" time for exercise)

As you can see, after it's all said and done, there are 12 hours left over for exercise, or 1.4 hours per day, and all I'm asking for is thirty minutes!

As a leader in preventive cardiology, it's important for me to "walk the talk." I know the benefits of a healthful lifestyle, and I see the ill effects of not paying attention to it in my patients every day. Yet my schedule is just as jam-packed as everyone else's, so I know the challenge of trying to fit in exercise. By practicing what I teach and making exercise a priority, I believe I can be more effective as a physician and scientist—and as a mother and wife. I tell my patients that by taking thirty minutes to exercise every day, we actually create time, because by staying physically fit, we have more energy, and we're more efficient. I feel much more efficient at everything I do because I take the time to exercise almost every day. Exercise also creates time that you can tack on to your future. Research shows that those who are physically active live longer. All said, none of us can afford *not* to exercise.

Exercise Strengthens Families

How do you fit exercise in when you've got a family to tend to? That's a common question, especially if your kids aren't old enough to exercise along with you. When our kids were really young, in the stroller stage, my husband and I liked to swim laps and run, as we do now. But money was tight at that early point in our careers, so hiring a babysitter and heading to the gym without the kids just wasn't an option. Our solution? We developed a system: While one of us drove our boys to the pool, the other ran to the pool. Then the one who ran to the pool played with the kids in the water while the other one swam laps. This system allowed us to both exercise and spend time with the kids. If your kids are little, you can take walks as a family while pushing the stroller.

There's so much payoff to having an active lifestyle that goes beyond heart health. Eventually, our active playtime together began to take on a life of its own, and as the boys grew older, we began adding other activities to the repertoire—hiking, cycling, jumping on the trampoline in the backyard and running together. It became a nice way for us to reconnect at the end of the day. (As teens, our sons now take great pleasure in beating us in a variety of sports!) Families need the bonding time that shared activity provides.

As might be expected, with all the time my oldest son, Matthew, spent in the pool from as early as nine months of age, he took to the water. And by age eight, Matthew was winning swimming competitions. It was good for him to have a sport, we decided, not only for his heart health, but also for the discipline sports instill and the self-esteem they develop, which can spill into other areas of life.

In fact, we wanted both of our kids to have a solid foundation for their self-esteem. So that meant our younger son, Mike, needed to have a sport, too. But we didn't want him to be in the shadow of his brother. Which sport to pick? Our mission was to find something he enjoyed, and better yet, if it was closely related to swimming, we could all stay in the pool area instead of splitting up.

Our answer was the diving pool. While Matthew swam laps, with one of us alongside to "race" him, Mike practiced in the diving well, with either my husband or me there, initially, to catch him. As it turns out, Mike is a natural diver. In fact, when he was a baby, he would wake us up every morning by jumping in his crib, his first trampoline/springboard. One day, before Mike could even walk, he actually catapulted himself and flipped right out of his crib (unofficially his first one-and-a-half somersalt). Ralph and I were stunned to see him grace our bedroom door—with a huge smile on his face, of course! Kids show signs early on for the sports they might be good at and enjoy. Look for those clues and foster your kids' enthusiasm. Don't pressure them to be the best, but to simply try their best and do what they can. Mike now trains year-round and spends his summers in China with the former Chinese Olympic swimming coach, Zhi Hua Hu. And like his older brother, he also dreams of making the Olympic trials one day. You just never know where a little play and a lot of passion will take a kid. We, as parents, can do a lot by observing and supporting their natural tendencies. All told, I just carried on the tradition my father initiated. I took my kids swimming and made it fun, and they took it from there.

Be a Healthy Role Model

According to recent government figures, the 15 percent of six- to eleven-year-olds who are overweight in this country (who numbers in the millions) have as much as an 80-percent chance of staying that way as adults and suffering from weight-related health problems earlier on, such as heart disease. The epidemic is likely to get worse before it gets better, unless we, and our kids, take action—and the sooner, the better.

But what are parents to do when faced with things such as vending machines in schools, the reduction of PE programs and the marketing of junk food to kids, things that are working against them and us? The old-fashioned answer may surprise you: set a good example. After all, you are your child's first role model.

When I was at the University of Michigan, I had a heart patient who was superintendent of a Michigan school system. Concerned about the rising rate of childhood obesity and the lack of physical activities for kids, he said something to me I will never forget: "Kids tune out 70 percent of what you say, but tune in to 90 percent of what you do." Set an example for your children.

If you're a parent, you're being watched, and your actions convey strong messages. Children watch everything we do as parents, a process that pediatricians say begins as early as one month. In fact, your influence carries more weight than television commercials or peers, especially when your kids are little. They notice and model things we don't even notice we're doing—from how we regard exercise as fun versus a chore, to our TV viewing habits, to how and what we eat. That's why I believe it's critical for parents to model heart-healthy behaviors, particularly in regard to diet and physical activity, as early as possible. The key is not to simply tell your kids what to do. Don't tell them to "have an apple," for example, while you polish off a bag of potato chips. Don't only talk about what's considered healthful and what's not, but also do it yourself consistently. If you can give that gift to your children, it's a skill they'll have their whole lives that teaches them how to stay alive.

You may have heard the expression that there's an athlete in all of us. Likewise, I think we all have the ability to act as preventive cardiologists, and the most important patient population in the world is our own families.

To help your kids stay in shape now and for the long haul, here are five health habits I encourage you to practice yourself to set the tone from the top down.

Play with your kids. If you want your children to get into a lifelong fitness habit, exercise with them rather than just urging them to go outside and play. Remember, the family that plays together, stays together. Make a commitment to do something active with your kids every weekend, such as hiking, going to the park or zoo, playing ball in the yard, walking at the mall, cycling side by side at the gym if your kids are teens, or even just turning on music and dancing in the living room. Family time is so important in and of itself, so if you can incorporate activity into it, it's a double bonus.

One guideline: the family friendly activities you choose should include those your kids can also do solo, such as swimming, walking, hiking, cycling and in-line skating. Non-team-related activities teach kids how to exercise on their own. In other words, your kids probably won't play soccer into middle adulthood, for example. But if you play your cards right, they'll swim, walk, hike, cycle or dance for the rest of their lives.

Have fun when you exercise. When you exercise—and your kids are around—make sure you like what you're doing. If you have a scowl on your face while you're on the treadmill or constantly check your watch, it conveys the message that exercise is drudgery. In general, be active every day and move for the sheer joy and power of moving. Besides the benefits you'll reap from physical activity, such as having more energy and less stress, your kids will take notice.

Similarly, to encourage your kids to be active, pick activities they favor. If you're not sure what those are, talk with them and be willing to experiment. Keep trying if an activity or sport doesn't work. And whatever you do, don't use exercise as a punishment or force your child to do something he doesn't like "for his own good." If you like to jog, but your daughter doesn't, don't force her to run with you. You'll give the activity a negative spin, and your efforts may backfire.

Curtail couch potatodom. To drive home the message that physical activity is important, it's also a good idea to discourage sedentary activity. Set a limit on TV and computer time, such as one to two hours a day, and abide by that yourself.

Don't be a stadium spud. As it is with many parents of pre-teens and teens, a complicating factor in our lives is having to drive them to all of their sports practices. It's terrific that they're getting exercise, but what about mom and dad sitting on the sidelines? It's easy to sit in the stands and watch, or to wait in the car, but why not get up and move?

We've learned to bring along our exercise clothes and use that time to fit in our own activities. After we drop off the kids at swim or dive practice on the weekends, we try to go running around a nearby track or swim laps in the pool ourselves, so their practice time is a win/win experience.

Working Out with the Physical Activity Pyramid

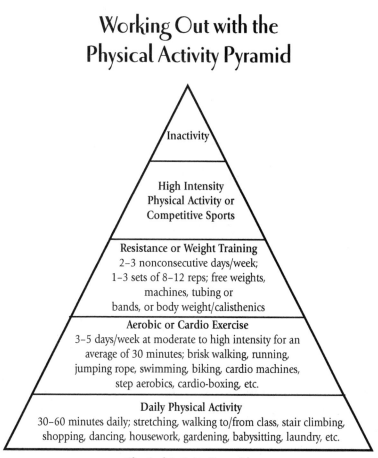

Inactivity

High Intensity
Physical Activity or
Competitive Sports

Resistance or Weight Training
2–3 nonconsecutive days/week;
1–3 sets of 8–12 reps; free weights,
machines, tubing or
bands, or body weight/calisthenics

Aerobic or Cardio Exercise
3–5 days/week at moderate to high intensity for an
average of 30 minutes; brisk walking, running,
jumping rope, swimming, biking, cardio machines,
step aerobics, cardio-boxing, etc.

Daily Physical Activity
30–60 minutes daily; stretching, walking to/from class, stair climbing,
shopping, dancing, housework, gardening, babysitting, laundry, etc.

Physical Activity Pyramid

With all the information out there about how much exercise you need and which activities count, it's easy to feel overwhelmed and confused about what you need to do to get fit and stay in shape. Enter the physical activity pyramid, which was created in the early 1990s by Charles B. Corbin, Ph.D., an exercise physiologist at Arizona State University in Mesa, just after the original USDA Food Guide Pyramid made its debut.

The physical activity pyramid is a graphic representation that can help you meet your exercise goals, whether it's to reduce your risk of heart disease or achieve a high level of fitness. The physical activity pyramid uses a tiered-menu approach to help you conceptualize and execute a balanced physical-activity plan. Its guidelines track with current recommendations for physical activity for health and fitness outlined by various government agencies and professional organizations. Each level of the pyramid offers visual suggestions for reaching your objectives—whether you simply want not to feel winded when you take the stairs or want to get in better shape for a softball league.

Level 1: Lifestyle Physical Activity

The base of the physical activity pyramid is lifestyle physical activity. This is categorized by the workout you get from your daily routine, such as walking up stairs with the laundry basket, strolling with your toddler, or getting off the bus a stop early and footing it the rest of the way to work.

Lifestyle activity is at the bottom of the pyramid because that's the level of activity we want everyone to do every day. According to the pyramid and the Surgeon General's recommendations for a healthful lifestyle, Americans should spend at least thirty minutes each day doing lifestyle activity, which can be accumulated in three ten-minute bouts.

Lifestyle activity isn't going to give you high-level fitness, but you will get health and wellness benefits and improve your quality of life, which includes reducing your risk of heart disease and obesity. It will improve daily functioning, like being able to carry a bag of groceries without straining. And best of all, they're activities every one of us can do. For good health, make lifestyle activity the mainstay of your exercise "diet."

If you are generally inactive, start at the base of the pyramid by adding bouts of daily physical activity into your day. Walking ten minutes to your car and back counts, as does playing tag with your kids. Very modest amounts of exercise are associated with substantial reductions in health risks. In fact, it's the law of diminishing returns. You get more benefit by simply moving (the type of activity you need thirty minutes of) than by adding intense exercise to an already active lifestyle.

Level 2: Active Aerobic Exercise and Sports

Above the base level, the pyramid tiers get narrower as the activities become more vigorous. Level 2 depicts aerobic activity and recreational sports for three to six days a week with moderate to vigorous intensity for twenty minutes or more.

These activities, which include running, jumping rope, swimming, step aerobics and cycling, will rev your heart rate and get you sweating. You don't have to do level 2 activities as often as level 1 to reap added fitness and health benefits. You can even use this level (level 2) of the pyramid to counteract a sedentary lifestyle if you simply don't want to take time during the day to, say, use the stairs instead of the elevator. Remember that before beginning any vigorous exercise program, it's important to check with your doctor. Depending on your age and risk factors for heart disease, he or she may need to check you out first to be sure it's safe.

To give your exercise routine pyramid power, build your activity routine on level 1, then add level 2 to your workout schedule three to six days a week, as you see fit, especially if you want to achieve a higher level of cardiovascular fitness and get added risk reduction for heart and other diseases.

Level 3: Flexibility, Strength and Muscular Endurance

The third tier of the pyramid depicts two separate types of exercises: Stretching—for three to seven days a week—and muscle fitness training—lifting weights two to three days a week at a weight that's moderately fatiguing, one to three sets of eight to twelve reps for each muscle group. Muscle fitness includes strength and muscular endurance.

Regular stretching and muscle fitness training helps reduce your risk of osteoporosis and injury. If you want to lose weight or maintain your present weight, you'll want to make a commitment to this level because strength training builds lean body mass, which naturally increases metabolism to counter weight gain. You'll burn more calories, even at rest. Because we naturally lose muscle mass with age, it's important to do muscle fitness training as we get older to maintain basic functioning. If you don't have access to resistance machines or weights, exercise resistance bands work well. You can even use your own body weight. Push-ups, for example, are a version of muscle fitness training.

Level 4: Rest or Inactivity

At the tip of the pyramid is rest or inactivity, which is recommended in moderation. Spend the least amount of time here. Of course, we all need to sleep, and relaxation is important to keep stress at bay. But it's best to keep moving and not sit for more than thirty minutes at a time by taking frequent computer breaks and building in as much activity as you can throughout your day, which brings us back to the base of the pyramid—lifestyle exercise.

Overall, think of the physical activity pyramid as a menu of options for being physically active over the course of a week. If your mission is to shed pounds, you need to increase physical acticity and increase caloric intake. All three of the first three levels of the pyramid burn calories and can be beneficial for weight control.

Three Keys to Your Heart

Here are three key points I hope you'll take to heart from this chapter:

1. **Experience the half hour of power.** For heart-health benefits, doing just thirty minutes of moderately intense physical activity, such as brisk walking, swimming, cycling, dancing, gardening and/or yard work, most days of the week is all you need. That's it. You can even break it up into three ten-minute segments. For weight management up the ante to 60 minutes.

2. **We can all easily fill up our day with stuff to do.** It's not about "finding" time—its about "making" time for exercise. We owe it to ourselves and our families to make exercise a priority because we will feel and be better.

3. **Be an active role model for your kids.** For your family's heart health, you can preach all you want, but the most important thing you can do is to walk the talk and set a good example by being active yourself every day. To keep your kids healthy and help them develop good habits, what you do is so much more persuasive than what you say.

Chapter

Food Is Life

"Our lives are not in the lap of the gods,
but in the lap of our cooks."

—Lin Yutang

Maintaining a healthful diet is as important as exercise to preventing CVD. Together, they're your first line of defense. Even if you're an athlete, you still have to pay attention to what you eat. No amount of physical activity will make us immune to heart disease or negate a poor diet. And, as I've seen in many of my patients, exercise won't undo years of a bad diet. In short, what we eat and how we prepare food—whether something's fried versus steamed, for example—can strongly affect our blood cholesterol positively or negatively, the propensity for plaque to build up in our arteries, and our blood pressure over the long run. To beat heart disease, diet is a key player, the foundation, really, of our CVD prevention plan.

But who has time to eat heart healthy when you've got a family to run, a job to do, your own life to lead and maybe even aging parents to take care of? That's the sort of question I hear from my patients often. The answer: you do, of course! In this chapter, I'll share with you what I think is a good system, and what I do to ensure that heart-healthy meals and eating habits become the norm for the entire clan.

Parent Power

As with physical activity, parents set the tone for their children's eating habits. To teach your children to eat heart healthy, don't simply tell your kids what to do. Orders like, "Eat healthful foods," or, "Have an apple," don't work, especially if you're scooping yourself a bowl of ice cream. It's most effective to eat heart healthy yourself consistently and talk to your children about what you're cooking and eating while you're at it. In our house, for example, I've been known to explain why I'm using olive oil versus butter, and why it's better for your heart. I swear my kids aren't listening, but then I'll overhear them say to a friend who has come for dinner, "This is healthy," and, "This is cool," referring to the olive oil. It warms my heart to hear how proud they are of their knowledge. Who knew my messages were getting through? I certainly didn't!

If you've got kids, it's never too early to get them started on a heart-healthy diet. According to the landmark Bogalusa Heart Study, which involved 1,474 participants over two decades, children with very healthy levels of blood sugar, blood pressure, weight and cholesterol were very likely to become heart-healthy adults. The study found that keeping those risk factors low throughout a person's life reduces the risk of all forms of heart disease, many cancers and other chronic health problems. Think of a heart-healthy diet as a long-term investment in your children's lifelong health.

Your Daily Goals for a Heart-Healthy Diet

While getting yourself and your family eating a heart-healthy diet, here's good news: there is no "special diet." It's really just about consistently making healthful choices about one food or product versus another. Everything you need to eat for a healthy heart is right in your regular supermarket. You can find it in the produce and bread aisles, the dairy department, and the meat, poultry and fish counters. In fact, I don't consider a heart-healthy diet a "diet" at all. Diets imply a special eating plan you go on and then off. We're talking about a lifelong nutritional way of living. Fortunately, it's easy to do when you keep these objectives in mind.

Consume at least five servings of fruits and vegetables a day. Look for deep-colored produce because it's high in vitamins, minerals and antioxidants, not to mention fiber. It's also likely to be a good source of folate, the food form of folic acid. Folate/folic acid and other B vitamins help break down homocysteine, a substance in the blood that has been associated with an increased risk of atherosclerosis. Besides helping to prevent CVD, folic acid helps prevent neural tube defects. Women of childbearing age need at least 400 micrograms of folic acid daily. Produce is also low in fat, calories and sodium, and contains no cholesterol.

Eat foods high in fiber. If you're like most Americans, you're fiber challenged. According to the American Heart Association, Americans consume only 15 grams of fiber daily. But if we got closer to the recommendation of 20 to 35 grams of fiber per day, our hearts and our overall health would benefit. That's because fiber not only helps reduce LDL cholesterol to reduce our risk of CVD, it helps control blood sugar to reduce our risk of type 2 diabetes, also a CVD risk factor. Eating plenty of fiber-containing foods also promotes proper bowel function to speed waste through the digestive tract. High-fiber foods may also help us to feel full with fewer calories to help control our weight.

On a heart-healthy diet, your goal is to consume 20 or more grams of fiber per day. In fact, the 2005 dietary guidelines recommend consuming three ounces or more of whole grains per day. In my preventive cardiology program, we call these foods "high-quality carbohydrates." Fiber, particularly heart-healthy soluble fiber, may reduce LDL (the "bad") cholesterol. To fiber up your diet and give your jaw a workout, think whole-grain breads and cereals, beans and legumes, and fruits and vegetables, all of which are excellent sources of fiber. More specifically:

- **Eat more whole foods.** At the top of the list are: fruits and vegetables, such as carrots, squash, broccoli, leafy greens and potatoes with the skin. Aim to consume five to nine servings of these types of fruits and vegetables daily. If you're eating out, choose entrées that come with a lot of vegetables. For dessert and snacks, opt for fruit. High-fiber favorites include berries, dried fruit, and anything with the skin, such as nectarines, plums and pears. Moreover, beans, peas and legumes are also outstanding fiber sources. For example, a cup of black or navy bean soup has at least 10 to 12 grams of fiber, which is about half the daily recommendation. Other ways to sneak fiber in: sprinkle kidney beans or chickpeas on your salad-bar salad, and opt for soups containing whole grains, such as barley or brown rice, whenever possible, instead of, say, chicken noodle or cream of mushroom.
- **Choose whole-grain cereals like oatmeal for breakfast or as a snack and whole-grain bread instead of white.** For example, order whole-wheat bread on your deli sandwich. One caveat: spotting high-fiber whole-grain bread products at the supermarket can be tricky. With a tinge of molasses or caramel food coloring, some breads, for example, can be made to look

like they're high in fiber when they're really made from refined white flour. In general, to choose a high-fiber bread or cereal product, don't go by color. Instead, look for these key words as the first ingredient on the nutrition facts panel: brown rice, bulgur, graham flour, whole-grain corn, oatmeal, popcorn, pearl barley, whole oats, whole rye or whole wheat. (Without the operative word "whole," as in "whole wheat," you may be buying processed white flour, which is made from wheat). And don't be fooled by phrases, such as "multi-grain," "7-grain" or "made with whole grain." They're often code words for nutrient- and fiber-deficient refined white flour. Or simply check the fiber content on the roster of nutrients on the Nutrition Facts panel. Choose breads and cereals with 2 or more grams of fiber per serving. Don't like the taste of high-fiber cereal? No problem. Just mix it with a cereal you like.

Consume less saturated fat. This means fat that's solid at room temperature, such as butter, shortening and lard. Saturated fat is also found in quantity in red, fatty and fried meats. Limit saturated fat intake to less than 10 percent of calories—that's 200 calories or 22 grams of saturated fat on a 2,000-calorie daily diet. Saturated fat raises LDL (the "bad") cholesterol. How can you avoid it? It's easy to eat heart healthy when you make the basis of your diet fruits, vegetables, whole grains, low-fat or nonfat dairy products, fish, legumes, and sources of protein that are low in saturated fat, such as lean meats, poultry, and beans and bean products such as tofu.

Of the fat you do consume, make it unsaturated. Poly-unsaturated fat should comprise up to 10 percent of your total calories. Monounsaturated fat can make up to 15 percent of your total daily calories. Think olive and canola oil, but in small quantities because all fat is relatively high in calories at 9 calories per gram. A high-fat diet, even if it's mostly good fats, can lead to weight gain if you're not careful.

Shake the salt habit. Your sodium intake should be less than 2,300 milligrams per day, which is about one teaspoon of salt, or less than one teaspoon (1,500 milligrams) if you're over fifty. Sodium raises blood pressure in some people. According to the United States Department of Agriculture, most Americans consume 3,000 milligrams of salt daily. And if you live on prepared convenience foods, which tend to have hidden sodium, you could be regularly consuming more than that. A cup of ready-to-serve soup, for example, contains 870 milligrams of sodium—more than a third of the recommended intake for an entire day. The best way to curtail salt? Cook from scratch. You'll have so much more control over your diet's sodium content.

Limit or avoid trans-fatty acids, aka trans fat or partially hydrogenated vegetable oil. Watch your intake of margarine and processed foods. Trans fats are found in unsaturated vegetable oils, such as soybean or cottonseed oil, that have been injected with hydrogen, a pressurized gas that changes the liquid oil into a solid and alters its molecular structure to resemble saturated fat. (Think man-made shortening.) Introduced into the food supply in the 1950s when convenience foods came into being, their main function is to give food products a creamy consistency or crispy texture.

Trans fats, which are also naturally present in low levels in some dairy products and meats, may also extend the shelf life of a product. And because partially hydrogenated vegetable oils don't become rancid quickly at high temperatures, they're an excellent medium for megabatch, commercial deep frying. But trans fats aren't natural or essential and provide no known health benefit. In fact, like saturated fat, trans fats boost levels of LDL (the "bad") cholesterol. But they don't increase HDL, the "good" cholesterol that cleanses arteries, which makes them doubly bad for your heart.

Trans fats are so unhealthful in terms of increasing the risk of CVD and other conditions that the National Academy of Sciences concluded in a 2002 report that "there is no safe level of trans-fatty acids and people should eat as little of them as possible while consuming a nutritionally adequate diet."

Taking Out Trans Fats

To help consumers reduce the amount of trans fats in their diets, the Food and Drug Administration made a ruling requiring food manufacturers to list the amount of trans fats a food contains on the label. (For years, they were absent.) Companies have until 2006 to phase in the label changes. But many leading food manufacturers have already removed the trans fats from their products, with no discernible taste difference to the consumer.

That's good news. Still, I urge you to take personal responsibility for reducing the trans fats and saturated fat in your diet, rather than leaving that job to the food industry. How?

- Check product labels. To spot trans fats, simply look on a product's nutrition facts panel. If trans fats aren't listed yet, double-check the label's ingredients section. If it says partially hydrogenated soybean, cottonseed or canola oil, it has trans fats. Steer clear, if you can.
- Get out of the fast-food lane. Need dinner in a hurry? In lieu of fast foods, opt for quick-fix options from your supermarket such as roasted chicken, steamed ready-cut veggies from the produce department and a potato zapped in the microwave. They can be just as speedy but infinitely more healthful over the long haul.

- Choose whipped, "lite" butter or trans-free margarine over stick margarine. Natural peanut butter, old-fashioned, stove-top popcorn, steam-processed ramen noodles, trans-fat-free crackers (check the label) and homemade baked goods are also a better way to go. Low-fat ingredient substitution, such as replacing whole eggs with egg whites or using applesauce instead of butter, works for many recipes. Even if you cook with butter, an artery-clogging saturated fat, homemade treats may ultimately be better for you than the commercial stuff made with trans fats.

Saturated Fat Versus Dietary Cholesterol

When it comes to preventing heart disease, there's another fat-related dietary goal (besides reducing trans and saturated fats) that's recommended by the American Heart Association: limit dietary cholesterol to less than 300 milligrams per day or three to four eggs per week, or if you are at high risk for CVD, less than 200 milligrams per day or two eggs per week.

Although dietary cholesterol, which is found in large quantities in foods such as eggs, organ meats and shrimp, can raise blood levels of cholesterol, especially LDLs, don't make it your main concern. Instead, concentrate on saturated fat. The body doesn't absorb and convert dietary cholesterol into blood levels of cholesterol nearly as efficiently as it does saturated fat. In fact, a diet high in saturated fat can raise your "bad" LDL cholesterol level more than anything else you eat.

Bottom line: While it's important *not* to lose sight of dietary cholesterol and eat four eggs a day, the best way to reduce or maintain your blood cholesterol level is to choose foods low in saturated and trans fat. When it comes to fat, make that your primary goal of a heart-healthy eating plan.

A NOTE FROM DR. LORI:
THE LOWDOWN ON LOW-CARB DIETS

On a heart-healthy eating plan, high-quality carbohydrates make up a majority of the calories you should consume. That's a concern for many of my patients who are trying to lose weight on a low-carb diet. Will a low-carb diet help reduce your risk of CVD? We just don't know. There's little evidence about the long-term safety and efficacy of any specific popular diet. Based on the evidence we do have about diet's relationship to CVD, the lifelong eating plan I outline in this chapter, which is in accordance with the most recent U.S. dietary guidelines for Americans, is what I recommend for a healthy heart. If you want or need to lose weight, simply modify your portion sizes so you take in fewer calories than you expend. Using a food diary can help you track calories. Writing it down forces you to face the truth—and reveals the patterns and habits that may be blindsiding your best efforts to eat right. Feel free to photocopy the following food diary page to record your meals and snacks.

FOOD DIARY

What I Ate	How I Felt
Breakfast	
Lunch	
Dinner	
Snacks	

Exercise Log

Daily Servings:
   Grains and Breads
   Fruits
   Vegetables
   Dairy
   Meat/Poultry/Fish/Eggs/Beans

Be Choosy

To help you reach the goals I've outlined for a heart-healthy diet (more produce and fiber, less saturated and trans fat, and less salt), I've devised a "Choose" and "Limit" list for each of six food groups. When you're grocery shopping, ordering in or out, or perusing the party buffet, select foods from the "Choose" list more often and from the "Limit" list less frequently. (Go ahead and copy this list, and place it somewhere you can't miss it, such as on your refrigerator.)

This choose/limit list is a great one for weight loss, too, which is ultimately a matter of calories in versus calories out, because the foods on the "choose" list are typically low in energy density, meaning they're high on volume and low in calories. They're forgiving. You can eat more of them and not blow your calorie budget.

Meat/Protein Foods
  Choose:

- **Fish.** Consume at least two 3-ounce fish meals weekly (the serving size is roughly the size of your palm). Not only is fish a good source of lean protein, fatty fish, such as salmon, albacore tuna and lake trout are high in omega-3 fatty acids, a "good" fat that may reduce the risk of heart attack. Omega-3 fatty acids make blood less likely to form the clots that cause heart attack. They also protect against irregular heartbeats that cause sudden cardiac death.
- **Lean red meat that's trimmed of fat and contains little marbling.** All meat, fish, poultry and seafood should be limited to no more than two 3-ounce servings per day. If red meat is eaten, it should be from lean cuts and eaten only in moderation.

- **Dried beans, lentils, split peas, peanut butter, tofu.** These alternative sources of protein are low in fat. Soy protein, such as tofu, also contains trace components of isoflavonoids, which may have significant effects on the risk for CVD. Studies show isoflavonoids may reduce the clumping of platelets and also be potent antioxidants. To spot foods rich in soy protein, check the label. The Food and Drug Administration has approved the statement that 25 grams of soy protein a day, as part of a diet low in saturated fat and cholesterol, may reduce the risk of heart disease.
- **Ground turkey breast meat.**
- **Chicken and turkey without the skin.**

Limit:

- High-fat/high-sodium deli meats, bacon and sausage.
- Liver and organ meats.
- Egg yolks. Because egg yolks are relatively high in cholesterol (approximately 213 milligrams per yolk), you can't exactly have an egg a day and follow a heart-healthy eating plan, which limits cholesterol to less than 300 milligrams per day. Still, you can have three to four eggs per week and do just fine.
- Anything fried.
- Heavily marbled prime cuts of red meat.
- High-fat ground beef.

Eating Fish When You're Pregnant or Planning to Become Pregnant

If you're pregnant, nursing or thinking of becoming pregnant, you may want to avoid eating some types of fish due to possible mercury contamination. Mercury, a metallic element that's naturally present in the environment and accumulates in streams and oceans, can harm an unborn baby or a young child's developing nervous system. The Food and Drug Administration advises pregnant women against consuming shark, swordfish, king mackerel or tilefish because they may contain high levels of mercury. You should also avoid feeding these types of fish to young children. According to the FDA, it's fine for pregnant women and young children to consume up to 12 ounces of fish (two meal's worth) that's typically lower in mercury, such as canned light tuna, salmon, pollack and catfish weekly.

Breads and Cereals
Choose:

- **Whole grains, such as oatmeal, whole-grain bread, barley, brown rice.** Whole grains haven't been stripped of their bran and germ layers during milling; consequently, they're higher in fiber and other nutrients than refined-grain products. Specifically, they contain heart-healthy soluble fiber, which reduces LDL cholesterol. Strive for 6 ounces of grains per day, such as a cup of cooked oatmeal, a cup of brown rice or two slices of whole-wheat bread. Choose unrefined, unprocessed foods that have been tampered with as little as possible.

Limit:

- High-fat baked goods, such as doughnuts, danishes, croissants, muffins, cookies, cakes and pies. Think of them as the treats they are, aka dessert.
- Granolas made with coconut or coconut oil.
- High-fat chips and crackers.

Fruits and vegetables

Choose:

- Four and one-half cups of fruits and vegetables daily, especially those that are dark green, red, purple, yellow or orange.

Limit:

- Deep-fried vegetables. Deep-frying adds fat and calories and reduces nutrient content.
- Cream sauce, cheese sauce and butter.

FLAVORING UP YOUR FAVORITE VEGGIES

To add flavor to vegetables without fat, try roasting. It's a great way to let the deep, rich flavors of vegetables shine through. To roast, just toss cut-up vegetables in a judicious drizzle of olive oil and pop into the oven at 400 degrees for twenty minutes or so until they're lightly browned. The high heat, which sets roasting apart from baking, converts vegetables' starch to sugar, imparting a nutty sweetness. Any vegetable is a roasting candidate—from mushrooms, eggplant and zucchini to tomatoes, broccoli and carrots. Enjoy roasted veggies as a side dish, tossed into pasta, smuggled into a burrito or incorporated into spaghetti sauce, meatloaf or rice.

Or try this delicious zero-fat option. Instead of roasting veggies, poach them in nonfat chicken broth and white wine with garlic, basil or tarragon thrown in for a flavor bonus. Just add vegetables when the liquid boils and cook for approximately five to seven minutes, until they're tender-crisp. To retain nutrients, keep a watchful eye on the pot, or set a timer so you don't overcook.

Dairy

Choose:

- **3 cups of low-fat or nonfat milk** or the equivalent, such as low-fat and nonfat yogurt and frozen yogurt, smoothies, "lite" ice cream, and low-fat cheese, such as skim-milk ricotta, skim-milk mozzarella and skim-milk American cheese. Low- and nonfat milk products are high in protein, calcium, phosphorus, niacin, riboflavin, and vitamins A and D and have been shown, as part of a balanced diet, to help lower or maintain blood pressure. In fact, if you're at high risk for CVD because of high blood pressure—greater than the optimal measurement of less than 120/80—you may benefit from following a particular eating pattern called the Dietary Approaches to Stop Hypertension (DASH) diet, which is low in saturated fat, cholesterol and total fat and emphasizes fruits, vegetables and low-fat dairy products. For more on the DASH diet and high blood pressure, see "Your Diet and Your Blood Pressure," page 163.

Limit:

- High-fat dairy products, such as 2 percent and whole milk, coffee drinks made with whole milk, light and heavy cream, half-and-half, regular and premium ice cream, whipped cream, nondairy whipped toppings, whole-milk yogurt, sour cream, and whole-milk cheese, such as cheddar, American, Swiss, Muenster, cream cheese, brie, blue, ricotta and mozzarella.

Another "Weighty" Reason to Get More Calcium

Besides helping to reduce blood pressure, a diet rich in dairy foods like skim milk and low-fat yogurt may also aid weight loss. According to numerous studies, the nutrients in dairy foods work synergistically to mobilize and burn fat stores while preserving muscle.

In one such preliminary study involving thirty-four otherwise healthy obese adults, those who consumed three servings of light yogurt daily lost 22 percent more weight and 61 percent more body fat than those on a low-dairy diet, which contained only 500 milligrams of calcium (not an uncommon amount in the typical American diet). What's the connection? It's theorized that on a high-calcium diet— 1,200 milligrams per day—you inhibit calcitriol, a hormone that sends a message to fat cells to make more fat and break down less fat. Conversely, when we go on a low-calcium diet, we release calcitriol. The net result is more and bigger fat cells. But getting enough calcium alone isn't enough. The other compounds in dairy work with calcium to nearly double the effectiveness of inhibiting calcitriol.

Fats

Choose:

- **Heart-healthy, unsaturated fat.** Use canola and/or olive oil, whenever possible. However, because all fat, including olive oil, is high in calories, containing roughly 120 calories per tablespoon, use judicious amounts to help keep your weight in check.
- **Salad dressings made without "partially hydrogenated oils."** These are code words for trans fat. Check the label.
- **Nuts.** They mostly contain unsaturated fat. Still, they can be high in total fat and calories, so go easy, and choose unsalted.

Limit:

- Butter, margarine made with partially hydrogenated oil, lard and vegetable shortening. Such fats, which are solid at room temperature, are high in artery-clogging saturated and/or trans fat, which can potentially raise LDL cholesterol and also reduce the "good" HDL cholesterol.
- Salad dressing made with sour cream, cheese and/or partially hydrogenated oil.
- Fat and gristle from meat and poultry skin.

Alcohol

Limit:

- Alcoholic beverages to one a day (women) or two a day (men). (Drink equivalents are 12 ounces of beer, 4 ounces of wine and 1.5 ounces of 80-proof spirits.) More than that daily amount may increase breast cancer risk in woman, raise blood pressure and increase the likelihood of alcohol dependency.

Heart-Healthy Checklist

	Choose	Limit
Meat/Protein	Fish Lean red meat Dried bean, lentils Peanut butter Tofu Ground turkey Chicken without skin	Deli and organ meats Egg yolks Anything fried Prime cuts of red meat High-fat ground beef
Breads and Cereals	Whole grains Oatmeal Brown rice	High-fat baked goods Granola with coconut or coconut oil Chips and crackers
Fruits and Vegetables	Fresh items ($4\frac{1}{2}$ cups daily)	Deep-fried vegetables Cream sauce, cheese sauce
Dairy	Low-fat or nonfat milk (3 cups daily) Low-fat yogurt Skim-milk cheese (ricotta, mozzarella)	Whole milk and cream Premium ice cream Whole-milk yogurt Whole-milk cheese (cheddar, American, Swiss)
Fats	Canola or olive oil Nuts	Butter and margarine Partially hydrogenated oils Salad dressing with cream or cheese Fat, gristle, poultry skin

Shopping Savvy

To help you make heart-healthy selections when you're grocery shopping, study food ingredients and nutrition facts and compare labels. In general, the lower the saturated fat, the better. Watch out for clever marketing traps. For example, something labeled as having "no cholesterol" may still be high in saturated fat. Moreover, fat-free foods can still be jam-packed with calories. Here are good definitions to know with regard to reading labels:

- **Low fat** means less than 3 grams of fat per serving.
- **Low in saturated fat** means less than or equal to 1 gram of saturated fat per serving.
- **Low cholesterol** means less than or equal to 20 milligrams of cholesterol per serving.
- **Fat-free or nonfat** means less than or equal to .5 grams of fat per serving.
- **Reduced fat or lower fat** is at least 20 percent less fat per serving than the original item.
- **Light** means the product contains at least 33 percent fewer calories or 50 percent less fat per serving than the original item.

The Heart-Healthy Plate

To give you an even clearer picture, literally, of what you should be eating for a healthy heart, here's a visual model of what your plate should look like created by my staff at NewYork-Presbyterian Hospital. Once you get into the habit of setting it up this way, you'll have a mental snapshot that will come in handy no matter where you're eating, whether at home, in a hotel room or in a restaurant. In dining-out situations, you may not have as much control over the portion size allotted to you, but you can take charge of how much you eat and in what proportions.

A NOTE FROM DR. LORI: NO FORBIDDEN FOODS

On a heart-healthy diet, there's nothing that's an absolute no-no. In fact, that strategy can backfire. If you make anything off-limits, psychologically you may begin to crave it. Even with kids, studies show that restricting foods they like leads them to be more interested in those foods and to eat them when you're not around to police their intake, such as when they're at a friend's birthday party. Their mind-set is that they need to get this food while they can.

Even I have premium ice cream now and then! And so do my kids. Surf and turf? You bet. But foods such as these are like the red velvet dress or favorite holiday tie you may have hanging in your closet—they're not for every day. Save them for special occasions or the odd night out. If that seems too stringent, okay—have a small treat more often. All told, you can enjoy snacks and sweets and other foods high in saturated fat sometimes, if you make sure that most of the time you and your family are making healthful food choices. It's all about balance.

The Healthy Breakfast-Plate Model

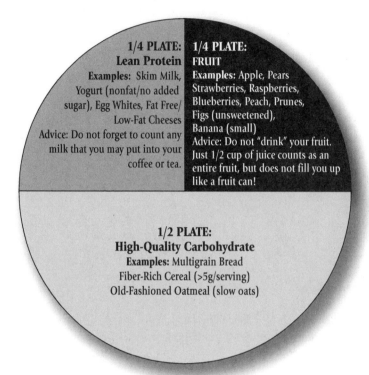

1/4 PLATE: Lean Protein
Examples: Skim Milk, Yogurt (nonfat/no added sugar), Egg Whites, Fat Free/Low-Fat Cheeses
Advice: Do not forget to count any milk that you may put into your coffee or tea.

1/4 PLATE: FRUIT
Examples: Apple, Pears Strawberries, Raspberries, Blueberries, Peach, Prunes, Figs (unsweetened), Banana (small)
Advice: Do not "drink" your fruit. Just 1/2 cup of juice counts as an entire fruit, but does not fill you up like a fruit can!

1/2 PLATE: High-Quality Carbohydrate
Examples: Multigrain Bread
Fiber-Rich Cereal (>5g/serving)
Old-Fashioned Oatmeal (slow oats)

Notes:

1. Oils, spreads, jams and jellies are "extras" and should be accounted for when tallying total calorie, carbohydrate and/or total fat intake(s).

2. If diabetic, check your blood sugar before each meal and adjust portions as needed.

The Healthy Lunch/Dinner-Plate Model

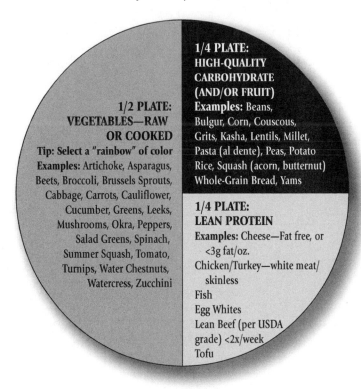

1/4 PLATE: HIGH-QUALITY CARBOHYDRATE (AND/OR FRUIT)
Examples: Beans, Bulgur, Corn, Couscous, Grits, Kasha, Lentils, Millet, Pasta (al dente), Peas, Potato Rice, Squash (acorn, butternut) Whole-Grain Bread, Yams

1/2 PLATE: VEGETABLES—RAW OR COOKED
Tip: Select a "rainbow" of color
Examples: Artichoke, Asparagus, Beets, Broccoli, Brussels Sprouts, Cabbage, Carrots, Cauliflower, Cucumber, Greens, Leeks, Mushrooms, Okra, Peppers, Salad Greens, Spinach, Summer Squash, Tomato, Turnips, Water Chestnuts, Watercress, Zucchini

1/4 PLATE: LEAN PROTEIN
Examples: Cheese—Fat free, or <3g fat/oz.
Chicken/Turkey—white meat/ skinless
Fish
Egg Whites
Lean Beef (per USDA grade) <2x/week
Tofu

Note:

It is important to keep track of the amount of fat that you add and to keep it moderate. It is always more desirable to use monounsaturated or polyunsaturated fat sources such as olive and canola oils.

Planning, Planning, Planning:
The Secret to Eating Heart Healthy for Life

In real estate, it's location, location, location. Similarly, to get into and stick with a heart-healthy diet, it's planning, planning, planning. I'm as busy as the next person, but I manage to eat a heart-healthy diet consistently and prepare heart-healthy meals for my family.

Here's what I do that might also work for you. The plan isn't perfect, but it does the job. I take one day, usually it's Sunday, to plan meals with the family's input, grocery shop and prepare entrées in advance for Monday through Thursday. On Friday, Ralph usually prepares fresh fish from our local fish market, so that day is taken care of. Saturday, we often eat out as a family or with friends, so I don't have to worry about that day, either. And on Sunday, we have more time, so we often have roasted a chicken or a turkey.

Preparing those Monday through Thursday meals all at once sounds like a lot of work, but everyone usually helps, so it goes quickly, and even better, it saves stress during the busy workweek. Moreover, we're usually all in the kitchen for a few hours together. It's another bonding time as a family, and over the years, my sons have become pretty good cooks. Cooking ahead at home prevents us from turning to fast food or eating out during the week because we're too hungry or tired to cook. It's old-fashioned, but home cooking is much more healthful for your heart in so many ways. In fact, I think that going out to eat is one of our biggest health challenges as a society. It's better to plan ahead, make most of your meals yourself, and get into a routine. Routine, routine, routine is also a key to heart health. If I didn't have this system, we would have a lot less control over our heart health because eating out doesn't allow as much control over fat, calories and portion size as when we prepare meals ourselves.

Here's an example of one of my weekly menus that includes a staple of recipes I tend to rotate through. (For recipes of some of my family's favorite dishes, see the appendix.) The dishes are hits with everyone, they're heart healthy, and because we do most of the legwork ahead of time, they're a cinch to prepare in minutes. In most cases, all I have to do is boil water for pasta, reheat the entrée and zap a side dish or two in the microwave—and voilà! Dinner is served.

Sample Weekly Menu

MONDAY	TUESDAY	WEDNESDAY	THURSDAY	FRIDAY	SATURDAY	SUNDAY
Veal chop; asparagus; low fat fettuccine alfredo	Skinless chicken strips and picante	Spaghetti with home-made sauce; salad	Lean steak; green bean casserole; roasted potatoes	Lemon sole or shrimp fradiavolo	Out-to-eat or take-out night	Roasted chicken; mashed potatoes; corn

Meal Planning for Success

I'm so committed to the idea of meal planning as the key to family heart health that I encourage you to do it, too. As I mentioned, I like to menu plan and prep all in one day. Ralph usually grocery shops; delegating helps make batch cooking doable. But there are all sorts of ways to get organized if that's not your style. You could pick one day to menu plan and shop, for example, then another to prep for the week. The key is to find a comfortable scheme that works for you. You could also make just one or two entrées to have on hand, then take it from there. Once you see how smoothly the weekdays go, I'm convinced you'll be a convert, if you're not already using this sort of system.

Your Weekly Menu Planner

MONDAY	TUESDAY	WEDNESDAY	THURSDAY	FRIDAY	SATURDAY	SUNDAY

The preceding chart can help you get started. On your planning day, just pencil in the menu for the week and make your grocery list from there. Then shop and prep ahead what you can. Feel free to make copies so you can use the chart week after week.

What About Breakfast and Lunch?

With my menu planning, I tend to focus on dinner because that's the meal my family and I try to have together. But breakfast and lunch are just as important for heart health and weight maintenance. In fact, studies show that eating breakfast, especially, is one of the most effective ways to prevent overeating at the following meals and mindless munching throughout the day. Its also really important for my growing, athletic boys to get about 500 calories in for breakfast, so there is no way we skip this important meal. Lunch is also important because it can give you the energy you need to get through the afternoon and avoid raiding the fridge and overeating at night.

Fortunately with breakfast, it's relatively easy to eat something healthful by grabbing a low-fat or nonfat yogurt, a quick bowl of bran flakes and a piece of fruit, such as a banana. If you're hankering for eggs, consider egg whites or egg substitutes. They're a nice alternative to regular eggs and can help keep your cholesterol in check. I'm always conscious about having many of those kinds of options on hand, so no one goes to school or work hungry. My oldest son likes to make fruit smoothies, and that's an excellent breakfast option, especially since he's so athletic.

Lunch gets trickier, especially if you're like me and tend to get busier as the day goes on. Many of my patients admit to having a hard time with lunch, as well, because their desk jobs keep them riveted. If that sounds familiar, I suggest bringing your lunch to work and keeping it in the refrigerator or an insulated bag. Prepare it the night before if you tend to be rushed in the morning, and keep a Post-it note by the door so you don't forget it.

I also like the idea of having kids take their own lunches, even if the school offers hot lunches. When you make your own lunch or have your kids take their lunches to school instead of buying them, you have much more say over fat content and calories. You're in the driver's seat rather than the passenger's. My kids have a salad bar at their school, and I encourage them to dive into that every day (with little added salad dressing). I also push nonfat milk or sports drinks instead of soda, which is a major contributor to the obesity epidemic in kids, in my opinion. I keep bottles of water readily available in the house also, so most of us go for that first to quench our thirst.

The recipe for a heart-healthy lunch has five basic ingredients: whole-grain bread, crackers, rolls, bagels or a tortilla; lean protein, such as low-fat cheese, lentil soup, turkey, tuna, peanut butter, roast beef or chicken; vegetables; fruit; and a low-calorie drink, such as nonfat milk or water. Here are seven lunch ideas you can make again and again (for kids, be sure to include low-fat or nonfat milk, if you can):

- Crackers and low-fat cheese, carrot and jicama sticks, an apple, and flavored seltzer.
- California turkey wrap (whole-wheat tortilla, turkey, hummus, sprouts), a fruit cup and bottled water.
- Tuna bagel (high-fiber bagel, tuna salad made with low-fat mayo and cucumber slices), grapes and nonfat milk.
- High-fiber roll, lentil soup, grape tomatoes, a peach and bottled water.
- All-natural peanut butter sandwich on whole-grain bread, celery, banana and flavored seltzer.

- Wasabi roast beef (high-fiber bread, lean roast beef with low-fat wasabi mayo and spinach), fruit cocktail (in its own juice) and bottled water.
- Chicken Caesar wrap (whole-wheat tortilla, chicken and romaine lettuce with low-fat Caesar dressing), an orange and flavored seltzer.

Don't want to make a lunch to take to work every day? Then grab a frozen entrée and stick it in the office freezer. (Check the label and look for those with 220 to 350 calories, 4 grams or less of saturated fat and less than 400 milligrams of sodium.) Add frozen vegetables to the meal to microwave later or a bag of baby carrots and celery to make it more filling. A frozen bean burrito is also good to grab and go. Or just wrap up leftovers from last night's dinner or order in a salad that features grilled (not fried or "crispy") meat with fat-free or light salad dressing and no cheese or croutons.

On a practical note, don't forget to keep supplies at your desk—napkins and plastic spoons, forks and knives, as well as salt and pepper packets—so you'll always be prepared.

Helpful Hints for Eating Out

On occasions when you can't eat at home, or don't want to, here's what I suggest to rein in fat and calories.

At chain restaurants. Zero in on the designated "healthy" section of the menu (which may be called "Heart Smart," "Lifestyle Choices," "Fit for You," or something like that) if there is one. The healthy-heart symbol from the American Heart Association is another menu icon to gravitate toward. These special sections—and more restaurants are providing them these days in response to

A NOTE FROM DR. LORI: COOKING WITH KIDS

Because I want my boys to learn how to cook heart healthy for themselves, I make a point of involving them in meal prep, even if it would be easier to just do it myself. Cooking heart healthy is a life skill I want them to take with them once they're in college and beyond. I know kids hate to be lectured to, so I'm always careful to teach, not preach, so they associate cooking with fun. In the beginning, we'd actually make a game of it. They'd guess, for example, how many baked potatoes it would take to match the fat in one french fry (four) to help them visualize what eating heart healthy really meant—and to see that they can eat so much more volume when they eat low-fat, when comparing calories.

When we're cooking together, I also tend to emphasize how eating well will help them build muscle to look lean and mean and boost their athletic performance. Most kids don't want to eat to prevent chronic disease. With my boys, it's easier for them to think about food as fuel—especially because they like sports cars—than it is to think about preventive nutrition. With Matthew, who is fifteen, I've also related cooking with dating. "You know, later on, when you get your own apartment, it's fun to invite girls over and cook for them," I told him, as we were puttering in the kitchen one night. "Girls like having someone cook for them better than going to restaurants. It's more romantic." His eyes lit up! Suddenly, he got motivated. Matthew thinks I'm helping him achieve what he wants rather than preaching—and I am, but I'm getting something out of it, too, and that's knowing he's picking up heart-healthy cooking skills he can use for a lifetime. For some of my family's favorite heart-healthy recipes, see the appendix.

growing consumer demand—usually feature items that are lower in fat, calories, sodium or all three. In fact, if a menu item is described as "low-fat," "light," "heart healthy," or "healthy," it must meet Food and Drug Administration labeling definitions. To give you an idea, "healthy" on menus means the item is low in fat and saturated fat, has limited amounts of cholesterol and sodium, and provides significant amounts of one or more of the key nutrients, vitamins A and C, iron, calcium, protein or fiber. Watch out for the old-fashioned diner's so-called "dieter's plate" (typically cottage cheese and fruit and maybe a hamburger patty without the bun). It is often an outdated version of what's considered low-calorie.

At chain and higher-end restaurants. Scope the menu for appetizers and entrées described as "grilled," "poached," "blackened," "with light coating," "roasted," "broiled," "baked," "steamed" or "drizzled." These signal that a menu item is comparatively lower in calories and fat because less fat is used during prep. If the restaurant doesn't take out the guesswork for you, you can do it yourself by focusing on menu buzzwords. Similarly, avoid dishes described as "fried," "lightly fried," "deep-fried," "battered," "crunchy," "buttered," "breaded," "creamy," "crispy," "stuffed" or "loaded," "cheese," and "bacon." "Sautéed" is another fat red flag because many restaurants sauté with butter. And don't be afraid to get your server involved in the selection process, or to ask for the sauce on the side or that your dish is prepared with little oil or butter. (Feel funny? Don't. According to the National Restaurant Association, 75 percent of restaurant goers customize their meals.)

Anywhere. Get a people bag. Eat only half of your main dish. The average restaurant entrée contains about twice the number of calories most adults need for a meal. Wrap up your leftovers, and save them for another day. Or even better, box or bag up half your meal before you begin to eat. When it's out of sight, you'll be less likely to eat it. For dessert (which is now often served in pasta bowls in some restaurants), keep it to five bites. Or order sorbet (it's nonfat) or fresh fruit, excellent heart-healthy options.

At fast-food restaurants. Think small or share. Don't "super size" or order a "value meal" unless you plan to share it with someone, because most contain too much saturated fat and calories for one person. Two adults can easily share one value meal and have enough food. Or if you're by yourself, order items à la carte, and get the smallest size, such as the smallest hamburger and the smallest order of fries. It may cost you a bit more, but you'll be less likely to overeat because there's less to finish off. Consider a salad or a chicken entree. Think twice about ordering anything fried or milkshakes, which are high in saturated fat and calories. Skip mayonnaise-based condiments and extra cheese, and don't empty out the salad dressing packet. They're all sources of hidden fat and calories. Get dressing on the side and add to your salad by first dipping your fork into the dressing, then the lettuce. You'll use less.

Getting Busy Kids to Eat Healthfully

One of the biggest issues we had with our youngest son, Mike, who is involved in gymnastics and diving practice after school, is what to eat on the go. If you have school-age kids, maybe you know the dilemma. Typically, Mike has twenty minutes to get from point A to point B, and during that time, he'll need to eat dinner. But how and what?

The natural reaction is to resort to fast food. That's okay once in a while, but it doesn't work regularly for Mike. Between his two sports, Mike is typically gone from at least 4 P.M. to 10 P.M. every school night. For his health and performance, he couldn't possibly live on fast food. So we looked for places along the route that offered more healthful options. We found a nice bagel shop, and their fresh turkey bagel sandwiches have become one of Mike's favorites. At his age and with his active lifestyle, he needs to eat every three to four hours, so this choice allows him to get through practice, then have a hot meal when he gets home.

Plan for Success

How will you make your meals heart healthy? What kind of changes do you think you need to make based on what you're doing now? What one dietary change can you make tomorrow? Write your answers in a convenient place—then stick them on the refrigerator so you never forget them!

Remember, the key to a heart-healthy diet is choice. Maybe we make twenty decisions about what to eat over the course of the day, such as whether to have bacon and eggs for breakfast or the bran cereal with fruit, whether to add butter to the sauté pan or olive oil, whether to take our lunch or eat out. We don't have to choose 100 percent perfectly every time, but if we can strive to take the better alternative more often than not, we'll do well. As far as our hearts are concerned, a single healthful food choice out of dozens can add up to a big difference over the course of a week or month when you keep it up.

For heart health, we don't need to treat food as a punishment or a reward. But we do need to choose carefully because there are lots of options out there. And as my son Matt would say, "Food is life." And that's exactly right. We should eat to live, not live to eat.

Eating to Live—Even on Medication

Over the twenty years I've been practicing medicine, I've had many patients initially come to me with numbers—their cholesterol profile and/or their blood pressure—that didn't look favorable. "If you don't make a change in your lifestyle, I'm going to have to put you on medication," I've had to say to them. Many were candidates for one, maybe two, drugs—one for their cholesterol and another for their blood pressure. At that point, many patients really get motivated and begin following the program I've outlined in this book. They start eating a heart-healthy diet, exercising for at least thirty minutes a day and taking control of their stress level. Maybe they even lose a few pounds. And it often takes only about a ten-pound weight loss to have significant effects on blood pressure and blood cholesterol.

Their efforts typically pay off. At subsequent visits in just two to three months, their numbers improve and the prospect of drug therapy is no longer in the picture. But then there are other patients who, despite stellar heart-healthy lifestyles, can't make their cholesterol and/or blood pressure budge. Their numbers remain abnormally high, due primarily to genetics. To prevent heart disease, these patients need medication, which I'll talk more about in chapter 8. But that doesn't mean they don't have to worry about their lifestyles, because diet has an independent effect on the heart and vascular system, even separate from cholesterol itself.

Diet affects blood pressure, blood vessel elasticity and the level of inflammation in blood vessels. So even if your numbers are good, or you're on medication to lower your cholesterol or reduce your blood pressure, you can't eat anything you like. You still should follow a heart-healthy diet because your lipid profile and your blood pressure don't tell us everything. As far as your heart is concerned, there's a lot going on behind the scenes that responds positively or negatively to what you put in your mouth. Your diet is powerful. Feed yourself well.

Do You Need a Multivitamin?

In addition to a heart-healthy diet, many of my patients ask me if I think they should also take a multivitamin supplement. When they first come to see me, I always have them bring a list of all the medication they're currently on, including anything over-the-counter they're taking. They're even asked to bring in the actual bottles so I can read the label on the spot and make an assessment. I've seen everything over the years, but I'll never forget one patient who literally brought in a briefcase full of vitamin/mineral supplements—a cornucopia of pills. When it comes to vitamin and mineral supplements, some of us think more is better and that because they're sold over-the-counter, they're safe. Clearly, this patient was a member of that club.

But over-the-counter supplements aren't tightly regulated by the Food and Drug Administration, so you really don't know what you're buying. Also, because so many foods are fortified these days, you can get too much of a good thing. According to a report in the *Journal of the American Dietetic Association,* if you're eating highly fortified foods, such as some cereals, energy bars and vitamin waters, in conjunction with multivitamins, you can easily consume 300 percent of the RDA for many known nutrients, raising the rare possibility of toxicity. I had another patient come to me who was taking more than a dozen vitamin supplements, who started complaining about unexplained tingling in his hands. When I asked him to stop taking those supplements, the tingling went away.

Overall, in my opinion, other than postmenopausal women who should take a calcium supplement and folic acid for women of childbearing age, we don't need any multivitamin/mineral supplements if we eat a heart-healthy diet. I'm not necessarily opposed to a multivitamin a day; some of us may like to take one for added "health insurance." If that's you, just know that it hasn't been proven to be harmful or helpful. But our diet has been shown to be a powerful defense against CVD as well as a host of other chronic diseases. You can't go wrong by putting your faith in food.

Your Diet and Your Blood Pressure

Besides influencing your cholesterol profile, your diet can also affect your blood pressure. Several studies, the first published in the *New England Journal of Medicine* in 1997, showed that following the DASH diet, mentioned earlier, reduced blood pressure considerably in participants with and without hypertension. Another study, published in 2000, showed that the DASH diet also reduces blood levels of homocysteine. High levels of this amino acid may increase the risk of heart disease, stroke and other vascular diseases. A third DASH study, published in 2001 that also controlled for sodium (salt), showed even more dramatic reductions in blood pressure, especially in those with hypertension.

Why is the DASH diet so effective at reducing blood pressure? It combines many nutrients that have been shown to be beneficial in lowering blood pressure. Those include calcium, potassium, magnesium, protein and fiber, as well as lower total fat and saturated fat. Each of those nutrients alone may not have enough impact on blood pressure to be detected in a study. But if they're together in a whole dietary pattern, such as DASH, their benefits may be additive and more likely to be detected. In fact, studies have shown that if you eliminate dairy products and just take calcium supplements, for example, you don't get the same synergistic effect on blood pressure.

Further, following the DASH diet may delay the need to take hypertension medication or even prevent you from needing to take it at all. If you're already on medication, it may help reduce the amount of medication your doctor advises you to take.

Although hypertension medications have been proven to be very effective at lowering blood pressure, having to take them isn't a panacea. Even if the medication you take lowers your blood pressure to a range that's acceptable, your risk of CVD is still higher than people who can control their blood pressure with diet and lifestyle.

Doing the DASH

The DASH diet is healthful for the whole family, and it's not hard to follow. On the 2,000-calorie DASH diet, you're advised to eat:

- Seven to eight daily servings of grains and grain products, such as whole wheat bread, cereal, oatmeal, crackers, unsalted pretzels and popcorn.
- Four to five servings of vegetables, the darker in color, the better.
- Four to five daily servings of fruit.
- Two to three servings of low-fat or nonfat dairy products.
- Four to five servings per week of nuts, seeds and dry beans.
- Two to three daily servings of fats and oils, such as olive oil and light salad dressing.

You're also allowed five servings of sweets per week, such as maple syrup, sorbet or gelatin, as well as one to two daily glasses of alcohol, if you like. Although the DASH diet isn't designed for weight loss, it easily can be if you reduce the number of servings you consume. Most of the food the diet features is low in energy density, which means it's big on volume and low in calories.

To maximize the impact of the DASH, lose weight if you need to and exercise regularly by incorporating thirty minutes of moderately intense physical activity into your day, such as brisk walking, swimming, cycling or golf (if you walk the course).

If you're serious about following the diet, it's a good idea to consult with a registered dietitian for support and guidance. In fact, according to a national study called PREMIER, published in the *Journal of the American Medical Association* in April 2003, participants who lowered their blood pressure the most had eighteen counseling sessions with a registered dietitian; they also kept track of their physical activity and food intake with a journal. Even participants who followed the diet on their own showed blood pressure improvement.

In fact, if you really want to take control of your diet, it's not a bad idea to align yourself with a registered dietitian. Every single patient in my practice sees Heidi Mochari, RD, the same day they see me—that's how important I think nutrition is! We never put them on a diet, but simply suggest the adjustments they need to make to achieve their heart-health goals.

For the names of RDs in your area who are familiar with the DASH diet, log on to the American Dietetic Association at *www.eatright.org.* You might screen dietitians by asking how familiar they are with the DASH diet or how much experience they have with cardiac patients, even if you're technically not one, because the nutritional issues of a cardiac patient tend to be relevant for everyone.

Three Keys to Your Heart

Here are three key points I hope you'll take to heart from this chapter:

1. **There's nothing "special" about a heart-healthy diet.** In fact, it's incredibly mainstream. The gist: Eat a diet that offers a variety of fruits and vegetables, grains, low-fat or nonfat dairy products, fish, legumes, and other sources of protein low in saturated fat, such as poultry sans the skin and lean meats. Limit saturated fat and trans fat.

2. **Planning is everything.** To make a heart-healthy diet work, plan your meals in advance, and cook ahead so you'll have meals on hand. That way, you won't have to resort to ordering in or eating out when time is short. I'm convinced meal-planning and organization is the key to long-term heart-health success.

3. **Get your kids involved.** Your job as a heart-smartiologist and parent is to give your children life skills they can use after they leave home. While you're preparing heart-healthy meals and grocery shopping, mention to your kids what's heart-healthy, what's not so great, and why you're buying or using that food or product. Even better, have them help you prepare meals. They'll be so much more motivated to eat heart-healthy meals when they've had a hand in them—and they'll learn how to cook, too, which is an important life skill for all of us. And keep in mind that your kids will never know they're "learning" if you make cooking fun.

Chapter

7

Health: Personal Priority #1

"Things which matter most must never be at the mercy of things which matter least."

—Goethe

I loved growing up in central New York. The changing seasons always gave me a sense of inner peace and excitement about what was ahead. But just like winters in Syracuse, change itself can be bittersweet because it usually requires letting go of something with which we're comfortable. Change is hard, especially when it involves lifestyle, because it means changing priorities. As Henry David Thoreau said, "Things do not change. We change."

As a physician specializing in preventive cardiology, I spend my professional life trying to help people change their lifestyles, their risk level and, ultimately, their lives. Change is hard for nearly everyone, and many of my patients have defense mechanisms to resist it. Some experience denial. They respond to my warnings with, "It won't happen to me," or, "It's not happening to me." Many of my patients, including those who've actually been diagnosed with CVD, frequently confirm this reality for me.

Denial. I'll never forget one patient, a forty-year-old mother of two children under the age of four who had such a major case of denial that I had to dig deep to get through to her. This patient, whom I'll call Patricia, had just undergone angioplasty, a common but serious procedure to unblock arteries. She also had two stents—wire mesh tubes—inserted to keep those arteries propped open. (Patricia, by the way, drove herself to the emergency room when she experienced CVD symptoms because she—like my father—didn't want to bother anyone.)

After angioplasty, cardiac rehabilitation was the next step in Patricia's road to recovery. Cardiac rehab, a comprehensive, medically managed program to help heart patients recuperate and improve their overall physical and mental functioning, usually includes education on how to modify risk factors, such as diet and high blood pressure, as well as a supervised exercise program. Granted, it requires frequent visits to a cardiac rehabilitation center for therapy, but it's worth it. Rehab can improve the chances of survival after a major cardiac event by 25 percent, which is sizeable. "You should go to cardiac rehab," I urged Patricia many times during her appointments, citing the 25 percent statistic. But I could see she wasn't fazed. Her life was complicated, she insisted. Cardiac rehab? Ha! "I don't have time. I've got to take care of my kids, and my mother is dying of cancer," she said.

Patricia was a particularly interesting patient because she had an Ivy League education and prior employment in a health care setting. She knew how serious heart disease was. Still, her head was in the sand about her own problem. I understood that Patricia's mother and her children were certainly important to her, but what about being alive? That trumps everything. What could I say to get Patricia to accept the severity of her situation?

"I realize it's hard for you at age forty to be losing your

mother," I began. "But have you considered that it's a lot more difficult to lose your mother at age four? That's what's going to happen to your daughter if you don't take time for yourself," I said. I could see from Patricia's reaction that she finally understood how important this was. As a physician, there's a point at which you get the sense you're finally, finally reaching the most intractable patients. Sometimes, it never comes. But in this case, I knew it had, and I felt a wave of relief. "Okay, maybe I'll go," Patricia whispered. Patricia went to cardiac rehab after all and started to walk with her children, which was a nice solution to her need for increased exercise. Walking allowed her to not only take care of herself, but to spend time with them as well. Still, let's not forget that by putting others first, she placed her own life at risk. By taking care of herself, she was taking care of her family.

Put Your Health at the Top of Your To-Do List

By keeping our hearts healthy, we put ourselves at the top on our to-do lists. I can't emphasize enough how we need to take care of ourselves first—above everything and everyone else, including our families and our jobs. You and your health should be numero uno.

In other words, yes, paying the bills is essential, as is doing a good job at work and taking care of our families. But we shouldn't be concentrating on those activities at the expense of our own health—and potentially, our lives. It harkens back to the goal of heart disease prevention, which is to increase your "health span," not just your life span. I once heard the concept expressed as, "We want people dying young at a ripe old age." In other words, we want to add life to years, not just years to life.

When we don't put our health first, it's called the "oxygen-mask syndrome," which Patricia was a good example of. It occurs when we don't feel important enough to put our own health needs—such as taking the time to exercise—ahead of our spouse's, our parent's or our children's needs and our other responsibilities. It's akin to the oxygen-mask demonstration on airplanes—when you're instructed to strap your mask on first, before putting on your child's, which feels counterintuitive to many parents.

Recognizing the Oxygen-Mask Syndrome

The subject of making lifestyle changes has always interested me, so I conducted a study to understand why it's so hard. I surveyed nearly three hundred patients, asking them what was preventing them from making the positive lifestyle changes they were prescribed to prevent heart disease, such as losing weight, exercising and eating right. The number one barrier for men was *lack of time* and for women, *low self-esteem*—aka the oxygen-mask syndrome.

Can you think of areas in your own life in which you put the oxygen mask on others before yourself, when you put the needs of others before your own to the detriment of your own health and well-being? If so, I encourage you to write down those instances and what you can do about them.

Example: *I always take the time to make sure my kids eat healthful meals, but then I skip breakfast or resort to fast food at my desk.*

Solution: *When I pack their lunches in the morning, I'm also going to make myself breakfast, which will help me manage my weight better.*

Putting Yourself First—Above Work

How would you need to change your life to put your health first? My career-driven patients have a particularly tough time with this question. They don't want to let go, reengineering their workloads to make time for exercise and other heart-healthy habits. Usually it's because they think they're too important and indispensable in their positions. They swear the company will fall apart if they don't put in eighteen-hour days. Granted, there are times we all have to work long and hard around certain deadlines. But if that becomes an everyday norm for you, it's a problem. Your heart will suffer. Your relationships will suffer. You will suffer. Yet I believe there are many of us in secret-suffering mode because, unfortunately, working twelve-plus-hour days is our national corporate culture. We think if we work harder, we'll solve the problem of having too much to do. Then maybe we can get everything done and have a little time left over for ourselves. But our productivity-oriented society just doesn't work that way. If we don't create time for ourselves first, and make that a priority, we'll always continue to find things to do to fill the time.

What can you do to buy more time for yourself and move yourself up on your list of priorities? To get my patients thinking about this concept, especially those who are filled with excuses about why they can't exercise, eat right, quit smoking and so on, I often say to them during their visits to my office, "I want you to shut your eyes and think of three things that matter the most to you in your life." I always give them a few minutes to think about it. Inevitably, they list some version of the same answer: their spouses, their children, their jobs or church, and so on.

My response? "You know, you can't have anything on that list unless you're alive. That should be the most important thing to you." It's an "aha" moment for many. "You've got a point," I've been told more than once. I firmly believe and repeatedly advise my patients that we should arrange our days, our lives and our priorities toward keeping ourselves alive above everything else. For some, that means delegating some of their work, so they get to the gym regularly. For others, like Patricia, it means going to cardiac rehab. For you, it may mean making an appointment with your primary care physician for a checkup or committing yourself to eating out less.

Let me tell you about one patient, Edward, who was, in my opinion, the CEO of the secret sufferers. He actually came to me to talk about losing weight, not for a heart-health evaluation. The owner of a small printing company, Edward talked fast. He explained that he really only had a few minutes for his appointment because he was so busy. But here he was in my office, and so I took the time to do what I normally do for any kind of preventive evaluation. I checked his blood pressure and tested his cholesterol and did other blood work. Then I started listening to his heart and lungs. When I assess someone's heart health, I don't just use a stethoscope. I also feel the heart with my upper palm (to avoid feeling my own pulse in my fingertips) to gauge how big the heart is. There's a location on the chest that's called the point of maximal impulse or PMI, which should fall in a perpendicular line from the left collarbone to somewhere between the fourth and fifth rib. That's where I should feel a nice, distinct pulse.

In feeling for Edward's PMI, it became evident that it was way out to the left, under his armpit instead of more near the center of his left chest. "I'm a bit concerned that your heart could be enlarged," I told him and ordered a chest X-ray and an echocardiogram, which is a procedure that employs sound waves to look at the heart muscle. It determines how it's moving and how large it is, just as an ultrasound takes a peek at an unborn baby during a prenatal exam. Indeed, these tests revealed that

Edward's heart was much bigger than it should be and was pumping oxygenated blood to his body at less than 20 percent (60 percent is normal), which signaled severe heart disease.

Long story short, Edward, a husband and father of two teens, had a cardiomyopathy—a heart defect—that was likely caused by untreated high blood pressure and years and years of a poor diet and lack of exercise. Frankly, I couldn't believe he was working eighteen-hour days. Edward hadn't realized how bad off he was because he never moved from his desk. Here was someone who wanted a new diet plan, but what he really needed was a new heart. Edward ended up on the heart transplant list. Only then did he realize he had literally almost worked himself to death.

A Lesson in Reprioritizing: A Christmas Tale

Evaluating what's truly important in life brings to mind the Christmas that our tree fell down. As the story goes, it was the first weekend of Advent. We promised ourselves this year would be different—there would be no last-minute shopping, decorating and card writing. We wanted to have a peaceful holiday season this year and to enjoy the final days before Christmas with our family and friends. I got up early that Saturday morning while our two little angels lay snuggled in their beds, then drove an hour to give a lecture on preventing heart disease. Luckily, the place where I spoke was a mile away from a brand-new supermall. I seized the opportunity to stick to my plan and finish my shopping early. That same morning, Ralph went to get our Christmas tree after surgery rounds, then spent Saturday afternoon setting up the fourteen-foot Douglas fir with his two little "helpers."

When I got home at suppertime, they had made it as far as spreading the Christmas tree lights all over the floor. Matthew, then age seven, loved the chains of lights that wound around the living and dining rooms, over chairs, under tables and between plants. Michael, then four, could barely contain himself from unpacking every ornament and running full steam ahead to show me how beautiful each one was. I declared an inadequate atmosphere. For the show to go on, "We must have Christmas music and a fire," I said. Ralph obliged and we worked until 10 P.M. to wrap the lights and ribbon around the tree. The children became too tired to help but too excited to sleep. We all finally surrendered and decided to finish the bulbs in the morning.

Sunday morning came quickly. We didn't quite "jump" out of bed, but we mustered enough energy to begin another round of tree trimming. Ralph put the finishing touches on the tree, and I began to prepare the children for church. We didn't have much time left to get ready, and the phone didn't stop ringing. While I was talking, I heard a sudden crash. And there it was, our beautiful fourteen-foot Christmas tree, the one we had spent the last day and a half decorating, lying on its side in the middle of our living room floor. Water spewed all over the carpet. The children came running to see what had gone "timber." Michael, with tears streaming, cried, "My bulb is all broken." Matthew shouted, "Oh no, there will be no Christmas this year!"

First, I laughed, then I cried. Ralph had to call our neighbor for help. They decided the only thing to do was to bolt the tree to the wall.

We dashed off to church in a state of disbelief. As we drove away, I looked back at our fallen tree in the window. Our top ornament was an angel, dangling with her toes pointing toward heaven. I reminded Ralph that I had told him to get a star. He wasn't amused. We made it to church on time, though somewhat frazzled. When it was time for members of the parish to request special prayers, I really wanted to ask everyone to pray for our tree. However, the person in the pew in front of me requested that everyone pray for Joshua, a little boy with incurable brain cancer. The tears welled up as I bowed my head and prayed for Joshua. I thanked God for reminding me to keep things in perspective. Our health was so much more important than having the perfect Christmas.

Mind-set Makeover

When you decide to cue yourself up and put your health first, lifestyle modification is often in order. You might decide, for example, that you're going to try to lose weight, quit smoking or improve your diet, all of which can reduce your risk of heart disease. But here's the thing about behavior change. Brace yourself. It's never as simple as, say, pledging to lose ten pounds as the televised ball descends on Times Square. By the way, research shows that many of us abandon our New Year's resolutions by mid-February. In fact, such carefree goal setting, however motivated at the moment, is a setup for failure. You can create a self-defeating pattern of making halfhearted vows, failing, then feeling as if that's evidence you won't be able to change your behavior in the future.

A better bet? Realize that sustained behavior change doesn't happen overnight. Researchers John C. Norcross, Ph.D, and James O. Prochaska, Ph.D, of the University of Scranton and the University of Rhode Island, respectively, followed thousands of people for up to two years to learn what works—and what doesn't. When it comes to behavior modification, they found that change occurs in a series of six methodical stages and that if you follow them sequentially, you'll greatly increase your chances of behavior-change success to help you get—and stay—healthy.

Throughout this book, I've suggested heart-healthy lifestyle changes to reduce your risk of heart disease. The stages of behavior change that follow can show you how to implement the behavior modifications I've suggested in *Heart to Heart*, so they become a part of your lifelong routine.

The Six Stages of Behavior Change

Stage 1: Precontemplation ("I'm just fine. Really.")

In this initial stage, you're not aware that you have a weight problem, for example, or you're not concerned about its consequences. You might even be denying the fact that you need to lose weight, because you've been demoralized by previous failures. But you're probably also aware of subtle warning signals that you need to do something. Your clothes are tight, for example, or your doctor tells you your cholesterol or blood pressure is high and asks you questions, such as, "What are you willing to do about this?" Your spouse drops hints about joining a gym. You don't feel all that great about yourself.

You know you're in stage 1 when: You make excuses such as, "I have a slow metabolism," or, "I come from a family of large people."

To take the next step: Don't turn a deaf ear to those signals—information is key. Suggestions: Learn more about the health benefits of weight loss by reading up on health and fitness. (You're on the right track by reading this book.) Write down a list of reasons why you want to lose weight. Most of us are successful in changing lifestyle behaviors once the desire for the change's resulting benefits (i.e., weight loss) outweighs the comfort derived from the status quo—staying just as you are. That's your goal in this stage, to fortify your motivation.

Plan for success: If you suspect you're stuck in precontemplation, knowledge is power. What benefits will you receive by making the behavior change you're considering? List them here:

_____

_____

_____

_____

_____

Review your list regularly. Maybe even put the list on your desk or calendar.

Stage 2: Contemplation ("I know I need to lose weight, but . . .")

In this stage of change, you're aware of the problem, and you're thinking about it. You're concerned, for example, about your appearance and are sick of wearing elastic waistbands. Or maybe you're out of breath when you climb a flight of stairs, and you finally want to do something about it. Still, you may have the desire to change, but not the confidence. This leaves you feeling conflicted and ambivalent. In this stage, you argue both for and against what you want to do differently.

You know you're in stage 2 when: You say things like, "I know I need to lose weight, but I don't have time to exercise." That's a common excuse I hear among my patients in contemplation stage. They've also been known to say, "I can't exercise because I don't like to sweat, I'm too old, I'm too tired. . . ." You get the idea.

To take the next step: Set benchmarks that force you to take action. For example, get the names of reputable personal trainers, nutritionists or weight-loss programs, and give yourself a deadline for making appointments—the day after your birthday or the due date for a big project at work, for instance. Also, sit down and take a few minutes to clearly define a realistic, measurable goal, such as losing 10 percent of your weight in six months by exercising at least a half hour every day and cutting 250 calories from your daily diet. Your goal should be that specific. Then plan a healthful substitute for the particular behaviors you're trying to eliminate. For example, if every day at 4 P.M. you run to the vending machine, plan a healthful, portion-controlled snack that you can eat without overdosing on calories, such as an apple that's stashed in your desk. Having a realistic and measurable goal, as well as a healthful substitute for the behaviors you'd like to change, is all part of the mental prep you need for moving on from this murky stage.

Relapse Rx: If, in stage 2, you hear the call of stage 1 (such as, "I guess being heavy just runs in my family."), get support. Team up with an exercise buddy or go grocery shopping each week with a friend who'd also like to eat healthfully. The support you'll get can be a powerful motivator. If you have other people watching your progress, you'll also be less ready to break that commitment. You can also start practicing positive imagery. Just visualize how good you'll look and feel once you've taken off a few pounds.

Plan for success: If you suspect you're in the contemplation stage for the behavior change you're considering, formulating a plan of action can help. What are the excuses you typically make, and how might you overcome them? Write your answers here:

_____

_____

_____

_____

_____

Stage 3: Determination ("I'm ready to go for it.")

In this stage, you're ready to take action and put your plan into play. You're finally prepared to lose weight, and you can prove it.

READER/CUSTOMER CARE SURVEY

We care about your opinions! Please take a moment to fill out our online Reader Survey at **http://survey.hcibooks.com.** As a **"THANK YOU"** you will receive a **VALUABLE INSTANT COUPON** towards future book purchases as well as a **SPECIAL GIFT** available only online! Or, you may mail this card back to us and we will send you a copy of our exciting catalog with your valuable coupon inside.

(PLEASE PRINT IN ALL CAPS)

First Name _____ MI. _____ Last Name _____

Address _____ City _____

State _____ Zip _____ Email _____

1. Gender
❑ Female   ❑ Male

2. Age
❑ 8 or younger
❑ 9-12   ❑ 13-16
❑ 17-20   ❑ 21-30
❑ 31+

3. Did you receive this book as a gift?
❑ Yes   ❑ No

4. Annual Household Income
❑ under $25,000
❑ $25,000 - $34,999
❑ $35,000 - $49,999
❑ $50,000 - $74,999
❑ over $75,000

5. What are the ages of the children living in your house?
❑ 0 - 14   ❑ 15+

6. Marital Status
❑ Single
❑ Married
❑ Divorced
❑ Widowed

7. How did you find out about the book?
(please choose one)
❑ Recommendation
❑ Store Display
❑ Online
❑ Catalog/Mailing
❑ Interview/Review

8. Where do you usually buy books?
(please choose one)
❑ Bookstore
❑ Online
❑ Book Club/Mail Order
❑ Price Club (Sam's Club, Costco's, etc.)
❑ Retail Store (Target, Wal-Mart, etc.)

9. What subject do you enjoy reading about the most?
(please choose one)
❑ Parenting/Family
❑ Relationships
❑ Recovery/Addictions
❑ Health/Nutrition
❑ Christianity
❑ Spirituality/Inspiration
❑ Business Self-help
❑ Women's Issues
❑ Sports

10. What attracts you most to a book?
(please choose one)
❑ Title
❑ Cover Design
❑ Author
❑ Content

TAPE IN MIDDLE; DO NOT STAPLE

BUSINESS REPLY MAIL
FIRST-CLASS MAIL PERMIT NO 45 DEERFIELD BEACH, FL

POSTAGE WILL BE PAID BY ADDRESSEE

Health Communications, Inc.
3201 SW 15th Street
Deerfield Beach FL 33442-9875

||||||||||||||||||||||||||||||||||||||||||||||||||

FOLD HERE

Comments

Perhaps you've actually hired a nutritionist or joined a gym. You're more focused on your goals, and they're starting to take priority over other things in your life. For instance, you may be willing to adjust your schedule to accommodate a postwork bike ride or aerobics class, and you've begun to modify the way you cook and eat. However, you may be cautious because the changes you've made aren't yet fully incorporated into your lifestyle. They're too new to feel permanent. You may be concerned about how to maintain your current efforts, for example, when the kids get out of school for the summer or the weather changes. Those are reasonable questions you can answer by staying flexible and amending as you go.

To take the next step: Reality-test all the changes you plan to make to get an idea of whether they'll stick around for the long haul. If you want to give up high-fat takeout dinners but don't have time to cook, make sure you stock your kitchen with low-fat meals, bagged salads, and fruits and vegetables each week so you have easy, healthy meal fixings on hand. (See chapter 6 for specific ways to heart-disease-proof your diet.) Similarly, if you're pressed for time but would like to burn 250 calories a day through exercise, find creative ways to incorporate physical activity into your day. Plan to get off the elevator early and take the stairs the rest of the way. If you're not a morning person, don't swear to hit the gym before sunrise; you're likely to hit the snooze button instead and scrap exercise altogether. Try to exercise during lunch or at night instead.

Troubleshoot so you can design a plan that's truly doable. All told, to increase your chances of behavior-change success, tailor your goals to your lifestyle, while also amending your lifestyle to your goals.

Relapse Rx: Develop a structure and routine. Know which days you'll weight train, where you'll do it and how long it's going to take. Jot down your workouts as appointments in your calendar at the beginning of each week so you'll be more likely to stick to a regular program. Keep a food and exercise diary so you can track progress and pinpoint problems. During this pivotal stage, also be sure to reward yourself frequently, so you'll keep up the good behavior. For example, after a week of eating lots of fruits and vegetables, take yourself out to a movie.

Moreover, you should also make an effort to control your environment so old behaviors don't tempt you. With losing weight, for example, spend time with active people and avoid high-fat restaurants, at least temporarily. If you do slip back into old habits—which is normal and an important part of the learning process toward permanent change—use the suffering that's associated with the slip as a learning opportunity so you can sidestep it next time. Ask yourself, what was it that caused the slip? Was it something practical, like going to the party too hungry, then standing by the potato chip bowl all night? Or something emotional, like the fact that you were feeling stressed about a project at work? In any event, once you've nailed what caused the relapse, dust yourself off and get right back to your regular, new routine.

Plan for success: If you suspect you're in the determination stage, formulating a plan of action can help. What is your specific plan to change a lifestyle habit? Write your answer here:

_____

_____

_____

_____

_____

Stage 4: Action ("I'm on a roll!")

In stage 4, you begin to feel good because you're actually doing something about your problem. For example, you're eating (and enjoying) lower-fat meals, controlling your portions and consuming more fruits and vegetables. You're also exercising for at least thirty minutes every day. You feel a huge sense of relief because you've found a real solution to a problem that has been zapping your confidence. One reason many behavior changers fail is that people dive in at stage 4 without first getting mentally prepared for change. If that sounds like you, turn back to stages 1–3 and make sure you're ready. Do your homework first, and you'll be more prepared to succeed.

Stage 4, while characterized by success, is no time to ease up, even though you may feel like it. To avoid reverting back to your old ways, you need to continue doing everything you were in the determination stage—planning, rewarding yourself and opting for your healthful substitute.

To take the next step: Learn to think on your feet in the face of obstacles. For instance, if a neighbor brings a fattening dessert to your party, accept it graciously—and parcel out the leftovers to guests as they leave. Another strategy might be to minimize the opportunities to eat foods you'd rather not. Don't go to a doughnut shop to get your morning coffee, for example, so you won't be tempted to buy a treat as well.

Relapse Rx: Fight the urge to fall prey to the "saint or sinner" thinking, as in, "I've eaten all of the chocolate cake, so I might as well give up." Continue to practice relapse prevention, as in, "I ate cake. Ah well. Now it's time to get back to my regular routine." If you're losing motivation, mix things up a bit and buy yourself a new pair of running shoes, or try a different class at the gym once a week. Set minigoals in your eating plan, too. Each week that you resist the pull of the snack machine at your office (or whatever it is that's throwing you off), reward yourself with a manicure or a movie—or my favorite, a trip to the day spa.

Plan for success: Formulating a plan can help if you happen to relapse into old behavior patterns. What typically causes you to fall off the wagon, and how will you handle it when it happens again? Write your answers here:

_____

_____

_____

_____

_____

Stage 5: Maintenance ("I did it!")

At this end-of-the-line stage of behavior change, your new habits are a reality. You've reached your goal weight, for example, and cleaned up your diet, and you feel strong, fit and energetic. Time to kick your feet up, right? Not exactly. In some cases, as with weight loss, you may be able to slack off a bit. But to avoid reverting back to your old ways, you'll need to continue everything you were doing in the action stage: rewards, environmental control, opting for a healthful substitute and snapping back after a slip. In other words, no matter how many years you've been driving, you still can't take a nap behind the wheel!

To take the next step: Fortify your motivation—take part in activities that were formerly only on your wish list, such as rock climbing or in-line skating. Buy yourself a new pair of fitted pants or a swim suit. You might keep a photo of the old you tacked on the fridge as a reminder of how far you've come. Look in the mirror each day and repeat, "I feel great. I look good." It may sound silly at first, but you'll get used to it.

Relapse Rx: If you've gained a few pounds, reevaluate what in your life might be causing you to solve your problems with food. And if you do slip up, don't let guilt—the biggest motivation killer of all—set in. Instead, forgive yourself, and start fresh at the next meal.

Plan for success: What rewards will you use to maintain your motivation? Write your answers here:

_____

_____

_____

_____

_____

Stage 6: Termination ("I'm at a healthy new weight—for life. Ahh.")

You know you're in this be-all, end-all stage when your former less-than-healthful habits feel as foreign to you as your new habits once did. At this utopian juncture, the problem behavior you're controlling is no longer tempting, and you're confident across numerous situations—at home, at work, in restaurants, on vacation or whenever. Congratulations, you've achieved a new lifestyle.

Sound too good to be true? It might be. For many of us, stage 5 (maintenance) is as far as we get—and that's okay. If you've reached your goal weight, for example, but still struggle with occasional setbacks, give yourself credit for all you've accomplished. Even if you never reach stage 6, you can maintain your new, healthful lifestyle by making sure your motivation doesn't flag. Plan to keep up the good work of habit change. For most of us, sustained behavior change is a lifetime of maintenance. The journey is the destination.

Relapse Rx: Revel in the new you, and make sure to continue rewarding yourself for good behavior.

Plan for success: What rewards will help you keep up the good work? Write your answers here:

_____

_____

_____

_____

_____

Change Is Hard—But Worth It!

Change can sometimes be so tough that it can actually make you angry. I often remind my patients who feel this way about having to, for example, alter their diet, move more or quit smoking, that it's relatively short-term pain (typically six months to a year) for long-term gain. Matthew, my older son, is a good example of how difficult it can be to adapt to change. When we first moved to the New York area from Michigan, he had to write a story about anything he wanted to as one of his first homework assignments at his new school. He was ten at the time. Matt wrote:

I liked Michigan. I had a good bedroom and a nice warm bed. But because we moved to New Jersey, I had to give up my friends and my swim team. And all because my parents' jobs were too easy.

[My husband, Ralph, and I had explained that the reason we were moving was because we wanted a bigger challenge in our jobs.]

After reading what Matthew had written, I began to agonize about putting him through such a big change at that tender age. However, I got an unexpected payback when Matthew thanked me for moving to New Jersey as we were riding home from swim practice one day. "This is the greatest place anyone could ever live," he said. Okay, it was four years later, but still, he had adapted. Despite the pain and the emotional trauma of leaving his past in the dust,

Matthew was ultimately grateful for having done it because he had personally grown so much, and he knew it. The move had been worth it after all.

Similarly, no matter what kind of lifestyle or health-related change you're trying to make, the health benefits you're likely to achieve in the long run will far outweigh any discomfort you may experience during the transition process. Some lifestyle changes, like losing weight, you may appreciate in a relatively short time, like in a month or so. One patient, Patrick, a bank executive in his fifties, told me he knew he was making progress when he could walk up stairs without being short of breath. This was after just two months of initiating a daily thirty-minute walking program and losing six pounds. Other habits may take longer. Another patient, Andrea, a fifty-six-year-old engineer, has been smoke-free for a year. "That was after a year of failed attempts, but I finally did it, which is what counts," she told me. "I feel so much better in so many ways now that it's done."

Any one behavior change that results in a health benefit typically helps prevent more than one condition. Weight loss, for example, not only helps prevent CVD, it's also associated with a reduced risk of type 2 diabetes and many forms of cancer. You'll get lots of mileage from your efforts. This isn't just about looking better. It's about feeling better.

A NOTE FROM DR. LORI: A SERIES OF CHOICES

Overall, in addition to considering and working through the stage of change you're in, I encourage you to think of prevention as a series of choices rather than a lifestyle overhaul. Each day, we make hundreds of decisions about what to eat, whether to walk up the stairs, what parking spot to pick, or whether to relax with a drink or take a walk after work. You don't have to pick 100 percent perfectly, but if you strive to make the better choice more often, you're on the right track. In fact, a single good choice, such as consistently eating a healthful breakfast rather than foregoing it, can add up over the course of a week or month. We learned early on that we must walk before we can run. A series of baby steps will get you to your destination. To keep up the good work, think back about the healthful choices you make each day—and give yourself credit for a job well done. You walked a half hour during your lunch hour? Good for you!

The Fear Factor

Change is about overcoming fears, especially of the unknown and unfamiliar. There are times we're more ready to try than others. I'll never forget when my son Mike was in a diving competition when he was eight years old. He had to do a back dive to be scored and count for the team. He had rarely been able to do it in practice, let alone in front of an audience. The following is a story, which I've titled "Chairman of the Board," that I wrote for him when he qualified to compete in his first national diving championship three years later. He taught me a lot about knowing when you're ready to take the next step and when you know the time just isn't right.

The air was deadly silent. You stood in quiet contemplation at the end of the long and daunting board. With your back to those who waited with bated breath, you were the one who had to decide. I could feel both our hearts begin to beat faster as we fought back the tears. You were only eight but had the courage of an eighteen-year-old soldier. Each passing second seemed to grow into a minute, an hour and then a lifetime before you decided it wasn't the day to set the butterflies in your stomach free and conquer the back dive. You didn't jump that day, but you would eventually succeed. You would do so in your own time and in a way none of us could have imagined. Diving isn't about the board or about what you've done. It's about facing the fear of what you might become.

So you see, each one of us knows best when we're ready. And trying is never failing. It's practicing for success.

Timing Is Everything

Overall, timing is important when committing or recommitting to a behavior-change plan because navigating new situations takes attention and energy. The ideal time to make a habit change is when your motivation is high and your life is relatively a clean slate. "I'm going to wait until after the holidays to begin my heart-healthy plan," one patient, William, a forty-eight-year-old real estate developer, told me. It was the holiday season, and William said he had several parties to attend. I agreed that was a good strategy. After you've been in a new job for six months or so is also a good time to put your plan in action.

Just as you wouldn't start out on a trip if really bad weather is predicted or traffic is bad, unless it's urgent, a less-than-ideal time for behavior change is when you're taking a new job, having a baby, moving, switching careers, starting school or have lots of social events to attend. So the best thing to do is plan for success by knowing where you are, where you want to be, and the best time to start on a journey of change.

Getting Your Loved One to Change

If you're reading this book to help a loved one reduce his or her risk of heart disease, you can still use the stages-of-change model to help. The key is to ask questions to figure out which stage your loved one is in, then apply the suggestions I outline to help him or her work through that stage. Start by stating a clear, strong statement that reflects the problem, such as, "The doctor says weighing 236 pounds is a major health risk. She says you're overweight," to clearly define the issue. Then ask, "How do you feel about this?" If your loved one (let's say it's your husband) is:

- Unconcerned, unaware, uninterested or unwilling. (He says things like, "I'm a big guy," or, "I am not overweight. This is muscle!"), he's in stage 1 (precontemplation). To help him change, try:
  — Suggesting that he learn more about the health benefits of weight loss by reading up on health and fitness (such as this book).

— Write down a list about why he wants to lose weight, which may boost his motivation. Does he want to feel better about himself? Keep up with the kids? Feel more comfortable in his suit pants?

- Conflicted, ambivalent or defensive ("I know, but . . ."), he's in stage 2 (contemplation). To help him be his own change agent, try:

  — Helping him define realistic, measurable goals, such as losing 10 percent of his weight in six months by exercising at least a half hour every day and cutting 250 calories from his daily diet by taking his own calorie-controlled lunch to work instead of eating out.

- Hopeful and has a plan of attack, he's in stage 3 (determination). To help him change, try:

  — Encouraging him to reality-test all the changes he plans to make to get an idea of whether they're doable for the long-term. Does he really have time to train for a marathon? Troubleshoot together so you can design a plan that's truly doable.

- Cautious, but can describe the specific things he's already doing about the problem, he's in stage 4 (action).

  — Help him anticipate obstacles. If he'll be going to a cocktail party after work, for example, help him foresee what's likely to be on the menu and how he can avoid overeating.

  — Encourage him to avoid "saint or sinner" thinking if he does overdo it. "Okay, just get right back on track," can help prevent relapse.

  — Be supportive. When he reaches his minigoals, such as walking to work each day instead of taking a cab, tell him you're proud of him. And make sure he rewards himself with something healthful for being so diligent. Recognize his efforts—just don't tell him what he's doing wrong.

- Confident, tackling the problem with new changes and seeing results, he's in stage 5 (maintenance).
  - Persuade him to take part in activities that maybe before he only dreamed about doing, such as playing racquetball or playing soccer with your kids.
  - Suggest that he post an old photo, a "before" shot of himself, on the fridge as a reminder of how far he's come.
  - If he's gained back a few pounds, talk with him about what he has been doing differently that might have caused it. Has he been nibbling more lately? Attending more business dinners? Upping his trips to the coffee bar?
- Hopeless, after trying to solve the problem, and no longer engaging in the changed behavior, he has relapsed. To help him get back on track:
  - Encourage him to keep rewarding himself when he does meet his daily health goals.
  - Make his goals yours. If he's trying to walk every night after dinner, for example, instead of watching TV, join him. There's nothing like having an exercise buddy to stay motivated.

Three Keys to Your Heart

Here are three key points I hope you'll take to heart from this chapter:

1. **Make your health your top priority.** From there, everything else should follow. Your job, your relationships and whatever else is important to you will be better off by this vital reconfiguration. By giving to yourself first, you're able to give to others.

2. **Recognize that lifestyle change is a process, not an event.** Because habits are so embedded, changing them isn't simply a matter of sheer willpower. It's a process that starts with mental preparation. To sustain the changes you attempt, make your lifestyle heart healthy, determine the stage you're in (precontemplation, contemplation, determination, action or maintenance), and work through the stages sequentially.

3. **Little changes add up.** Small, positive and consistent diet and exercise adjustments can add up to big benefits. To make your lifestyle heart healthy, don't overhaul it. Instead, change it by making one small positive choice at a time. Even something as simple as adding skim milk instead of cream to your morning coffee will do your heart good.

Chapter

When Lifestyle Isn't Enough: Managing Medication

"For so it must be, and help me do my part."

—A Tibetan master

Over the years, I've had many patients who, based on their risk factors for CVD, were candidates for one or more medications to bring their cholesterol and blood pressure within normal limits. Once they got wind that drugs might be in their future, however, they got motivated to improve their lifestyles and get with the heart-healthy program I've outlined throughout this book regarding diet, exercise, weight-loss and managing stress level. And within six months or so, their numbers improved dramatically.

Maryanne, a fifty-four-year-old retail executive, was one such patient who lost thirty-five pounds over the course of eighteen months by cutting calories and adding more fruits, vegetables, whole grains and fish to her diet, while limiting saturated fat. "I also started exercising every day for at least thirty minutes, just like you're supposed to," she said, proudly. Her efforts paid off. Maryanne's cholesterol and blood pressure levels began to drop within a few months of implementing her new routine, settling at healthy, optimal levels. Like many of my patients, Maryanne escaped the danger zone without medication, and I anticipate she'll stay there, provided she continues following a heart-healthy lifestyle.

But other patients, try as they might to bring their numbers within normal limits through diet and exercise, need more than lifestyle measures to reduce their CVD risk. Due to their genetics, they need medication to reach their goals. If you or a loved one falls into that group, take heart. You're far from alone. The latest national guidelines have nearly tripled the number of Americans who may qualify for cholesterol-reducing and other CVD drugs to almost one-fifth of all adults. Don't fret. Needing medication isn't a "failure," as some of my patients suggest to me during their office visits. Genetics can be powerful factors to overcome. Fortunately, several drugs have been proven to sharply reduce cholesterol and/or blood pressure levels beyond what lifestyle steps can achieve.

From Ann Arbor to Russia with Love

Having access to these lifesaving medications is truly a boon, especially when you consider that the citizens of some countries, like Russia, don't have the same advantages. In fact, Russia has the highest rate of heart disease in the world. That much my husband, Ralph, who is a pediatric cardiac surgeon, and I knew when we traveled there with two colleagues, Dr. Steven Werns, an interventional cardiologist, and Eric Jenkins, a University of Michigan

Health Systems perfusionist, in 1998, when I was the director of preventive cardiology research and educational programs at the University of Michigan in Ann Arbor. Our trip was a humanitarian aid medical relief mission sponsored by AmeriCares. The following account of our trip was published in the *American Journal of Cardiology* (1998 Vol 81 May 1).

From the moment we arrived in St. Petersburg, formerly known as Leningrad, it became apparent that Russia was a country dying on the vine. The cardiovascular disease epidemic is so extensive that the death rate in Russia now exceeds the birth rate. The price of the new-found political freedom has been devastating poverty; many Russians are dying from a lack of health care, food and shelter.

The head of the Cardiovascular Institute in Russia met us at the airport and apologized that the director of the cardiac cath lab could not join us because he had just died of heart disease. He insisted on carrying our bags himself, and we soon learned it was because our driver had also recently suffered a heart attack. In Russia, it's common for those who are lucky enough to survive a heart attack to return to work immediately because of the poor economic situation.

Our hotel was situated next to the battleship *Aurora*, which in grander days fired the first shot of the Bolshevik Revolution. Today, its gray decks sit barely noticeable against the dismal and deteriorating banks of the Neva River, which were literally built with human skeletons by Peter the Great.

The medical situation was just as desperate. We began our work at St. George's Hospital, a city hospital with dirt floors and crumbling walls. The team was immediately separated and put to work. I was informed what I could and could not talk about in my medical lectures. The head of cardiology asked me not to talk about cholesterol-lowering drugs because they had recently had a lecture on the topic, but I eventually realized that it was because no one could afford the drugs. It's too depressing for them to hear about things they can't have. During hospital rounds, I observed that the Russian physicians rely much more heavily upon clinical skills and experience rather than ancillary diagnostic tools. Confirmatory tests and procedures are extremely expensive and nearly impossible to obtain. The Western medicine obsession to treat based on the results of clinical trials ("evidence-based medicine") seems a bit foolish to their culture. They believe that no individual patient is exactly like the average subject in a research study. They explained that to generalize in such a way would be analogous to giving antibiotics to an entire floor of patients based on their average temperature.

Promoting the concept of preventive cardiology in St. Petersburg was challenging. Most of the patients I saw with heart disease were smoking in their rooms. One Russian colleague called the exporting of cigarettes "American aggression against the Russians." His sentiment was well founded since in a one-block radius of the famous Nevsky Prospect we counted fourteen advertisements for tobacco, not to mention the larger-than-life Marlboro man plastered on the building next to our hotel. Physical activity can be dangerous to your health as there is no emission control for automobiles, and the air is polluted. The water is also not safe to drink or swim in. The young physicians and medical students are quite interested in prevention despite the rather grim situation. They believe there will be a different Russia someday and that it's important for them to understand strategies to prevent heart disease. They want to be well prepared to practice prevention when the economic situation improves.

The interventional team, including Ralph, Steve and Eric, was on their own mission impossible—a situation quite familiar to Russian surgeons and cardiologists. Russian doctors are literally asked to do everything with nothing, and for that matter, for next to nothing. The average salary for a Russian physician is less than $200 a month, and they are often not paid for several months. They frequently have to reuse catheters and surgical tubing because they are in short supply.

Equipment is old and often requires creativity to get the job done. AmeriCares sent several million dollars in supplies with us so we would be able to offer necessary surgical items to patients who wouldn't otherwise be able to have an operation. The expectation in Russia is that if you're admitted to a hospital, you must pay for your medicine and supplies, and you must bring your own sheets and food. No wonder most of the beds were empty. We were able to provide assistance to some of those who made the trek to see us. We were worried it might only be the privileged, but then we heard stories of those who had spent their entire savings for a trip to see the American doctors. It was sad to turn away some who just couldn't be saved, and we wished they hadn't spent their precious few rubles to come to St. Petersburg, but part of our mission was to train Russian physicians and surgeons, as well.

There was one boy in particular who left a lasting impression on us all. He was seven years old—the same age as our older son, Matthew, at the time. He had a congenital abnormality of the heart; his prognosis was less than one year to live without surgery. Ralph agreed that he was a good surgical candidate, and when he insisted on talking to the mother before surgery, the Russian surgeons were quite upset. It was not their practice to talk to families. The mother appeared nervous but appreciative throughout the dialogue mediated by the translator. She had traveled over six hundred miles to give her boy his one chance and used the entire family savings for the trip.

When the surgery was complete, Ralph met the mother outside the recovery room to let her know that her son would be fine. She tried to hug him and said a few awkward words of thanks. She went back to her son's side, and Ralph turned to leave. A few moments later the translator yelled down the hall to wait. The mother affectionately handed Ralph a tiny green ceramic frog. It is a popular item in Russia, akin to something from our Cracker Jack boxes. It was the only toy her son had, and she wanted Ralph to have it as a token of her appreciation.

The global health care crisis of cardiovascular disease can seem so overwhelming that I often wonder how it could possibly be impacted. Then I remember a little boy in a country with eleven time zones, halfway around the world, who doesn't have any toys—but he does have a heart.

The experience underscored for me how lucky we are if we're born with a good heart, and how important it is to keep it that way.

[Reprinted from *The American Journal of Cardiology,* Vol. 81, May 1, 1998.]

Drugs Demystified

Are you a candidate for drug therapy? This chapter will help you determine that. If you're already on CVD medication, consider using this chapter to continue a dialogue with your physician. Don't assume your doctor has read up on the latest guidelines and will update your drug regimen as needed. A little proactive prodding may be necessary. A growing body of research suggests that those already taking prescription drugs to reduce cholesterol and/or blood pressure may not be receiving optimal benefit because they aren't prescribed at adequate doses to reduce cholesterol levels or patients don't take their medicine regularly.

Indeed, if your doctor prescribes one or more medications to help you control your blood pressure or cholesterol levels, it can be daunting at first. And confusing. After all, because the progression of CVD is often asymptomatic, you may not feel "sick." And because you don't feel bad in the first place, these drugs won't necessarily make you feel better. Under the conventional paradigm, when you're sick, you take medicine, and you recover. CVD preventive drugs just don't fit that model. Some CVD drugs may even have side effects, although in studies involving thousands, they're relatively rare. Most CVD drugs are well tolerated. Nonetheless, you probably won't get the immediate sense of relief you do from, say, taking a remedy to abate a sore throat. "Do I really have to take them?" my patients often ask, incredulously. Yes, you do! Ineffectual though they may seem, CVD medications are like janitors on the 24/7 shift, silently performing the important job of keeping your arteries clear or your blood pressure in a safe range, so you can go about your life without a hitch.

Minding Your Meds

To help yourself take your medication as prescribed, you need to feel comfortable with your doctor's recommendations and understand what the medications you're taking are and what they're for. That's why I always have my patients learn the names of all the medications they're recommended, the doses, their purposes and their possible side effects. When you partner with your doctor and have a baseline of information, you'll be more likely to take your medication as directed, which can save your life or that of a loved one, if medication is part of his or her CVD prevention program.

Compliance is key. Yet I've been surprised at the number of the intelligent patients who are referred to me who have no idea what medications they're on. Kathy, a top-level executive at a brokerage firm, was among them. At her first visit, I was shocked to hear that she didn't know the brand or dose of her cholesterol medication. She just knew she was on a cholesterol pill—that was it. To make matters worse, she wasn't even at her goal level. What was up? From our conversations, I got the sense that Kathy delegated nearly everything to her administrative assistant. For stress management, delegating some of your workload can be beneficial. Still, I told Kathy that her health was one thing she couldn't and shouldn't outsource. I gave her a homework assignment to memorize her medications. After that, her cholesterol profile began to improve. Coincidence? I think not!

When lifestyle isn't enough to reduce risk factors, medication management is an important part of a CVD prevention program. Here's a rundown of some of the most commonly prescribed drugs for CVD prevention for those who fall into the high-risk and intermediate-risk categories. In addition to helping prevent CVD, these drugs are also recognized as the standard of optimal care for patients who arrive at the hospital with symptoms of possible heart attack, such as chest pain (angina), or other clinical signs, including irregular readings on an electrocardiograph. Any one or more of these drugs are likely to be prescribed upon discharge. Please remember, though, that no list can be comprehensive. Get all the facts from your doctor.

Common CVD Drugs

Medication	Generic Name (Brand Name)	Possible Cardio-protective Effects	Possible Side Effects
Angiotensin-Converting Enzyme (ACE) Inhibitors	benazepril (Lotensin), captopril (Capoten), enalapril (Vasotec), fosinopril (Monopril), lisinopril (Prinivil, Zestril), moexipril (Univasc), perindopril (Aceon), quinapril (Accupril), ramipril (Altace), trandolapril (Mavik)	Reduces blood pressure by preventing the body from producing angiotensin II, a substance in the blood that causes vessels to narrow and raises blood pressure	Chronic, dry cough; kidney problems; weakness or dizziness; skin rashes; altered sense of taste; high potassium levels
Angiotensin Receptor Blockers (ARBs)	candesartan (Atacand), eprosartan (Teveten), irbesartan (Avalide, Avapro), losartan (Cozaar, Hyzaar), olmesartan (Benicar), telmisartan (Micardis), valsartan (Diovan)	ARBs reduce blood pressure by binding to angiotensin II receptors, which may otherwise cause small blood vessels to constrict	Kidney problems; high potassium, low blood pressure; fatigue; gastrointestinal upset
Aspirin	Brand names: Bayer, Bufferin, Halfprin, St. Joseph	Reduces blood clot formation by making platelets less likely to stick together	Gastrointestinal bleeding and increased risk of hemorrhagic stroke (bleeding into the brain)

Medication	Generic Name (Brand Name)	Possible Cardio-protective Effects	Possible Side Effects
Aldosterone Receptor Blockade	triamterene (Pyrenium)	Lowers blood pressure by blocking the action of the hormone aldosterone, which helps regulate blood pressure. Also reduces the amount of fluid in the body without causing loss of potassium.	Heart arrhythmias, shortness of breath, fatigue, confusion, weakness, numbness or tingling
Selective Alpha-1-Adrenergic Blockers	doxazosin (Cardura) prazosin (Minipress) terazosin (Hytrin)	Reduces blood pressure by causing blood vessels to relax and expand by blocking prostaglandins.	Vivid dreams, dizziness or drowsiness, weakness, fatigue, nausea, vomiting, diarrhea, constipation, abdominal pain or decreased appetite, fluid retention or slight weight gain, joint or muscle aches, increased urination

Medication	Generic Name (Brand Name)	Possible Cardio-protective Effects	Possible Side Effects
Beta-adrenergic receptor blockers (Beta-blockers)	acebutolol (Sectral), atenolol (Tenormin), betaxolol (Kerlone), bisoprolol (Zebeta), carteolol (Cartrol), carvedilol (Coreg), labetalol (Normodyne, Trandate), metoprolol (Lopressor, Toprol XL), nadolol (Corgard), penbutolol (Levatol), pindolol (Visken), propranolol (Inderal), sotalol (Betapace AF), timolol (Blocadren)	Lowers blood pressure by blocking the effects of adrenaline, decrease heart rate and cardiac output	Sneezing, congestion, itching, skin rashes, slow heart rate, drowsiness, weakness, fatigue, increased sensitivity to cold, headache or ringing ears, fainting, depression, reduced sex drive, diarrhea, constipation or nausea, low blood pressure
Bile Acid Binding Resins	cholestyramine (Questran), colestipol (Colestid), colesevelam (Welchol)	Helps lower cholesterol levels in the blood, specifically LDL cholesterol and triglycerides, while simultaneously raising HDL cholesterol by altering the way the body processes cholesterol	Constipation, stomach irritation, diarrhea, heartburn, dizziness, gas, headache

Medication	Generic Name (Brand Name)	Possible Cardio-protective Effects	Possible Side Effects
Calcium Channel Blockers	amlodipine (Norvasc), bepridil (Vascor), diltiazem (Cardizem, Cartia XT, Dilacor XR, Diltia XT, Tiazac), felodipine (Plendil), isradipine (DynaCir), nicardipine (Cardene), nifedipine (Adalat CC, Procardi), nimodipine (Nimotop), nisoldipine (Sular), verapamil (Calan, Covera HS, Isoptin, Verelan)	Helps reduce blood pressure by preventing the flow of calcium ions to the muscle cells of the heart and blood vessels, causing them to widen and relax	Headache, edema (swelling) in the lower legs, constipation, fatigue, stomach discomfort, low blood pressure, slow heart rate, impotence
Cholesterol Absorption Inhibitor	Ezetimibe (Zetia)	Reduces the amount of total and LDL cholesterol in the blood by blocking the cholesterol the body absorbs in the small intestine.	Abdominal pain, diarrhea, fatigue, muscle aches

Medication	Generic Name (Brand Name)	Possible Cardio-protective Effects	Possible Side Effects
Combination Medications	atorvastatin/amlodipine (Caduet), ezetimibe/simvastatin (Vytorin), niacin/lovastatin (Advicor)	**Caduet:** Helps reduce blood pressure by relaxing (widening) blood vessels and reduces LDL cholesterol and triglycerides and modestly raises HDL cholesterol **Vytorin:** Helps block the cholesterol that comes from food and reduces the cholesterol the body makes to lower LDL, total cholesterol and triglycerides and raise HDL **Advicor:** Helps reduce LDL and triglycerides and raise HDL cholesterol in the blood	**Vytorin:** headache, muscle pain, inflammation of the pancreas, gallbladder, gallstones, nausea **Advicor:** Flushing, rapid heartbeat, liver problems, muscle pain, dizziness, stomach upset, diarrhea **Caduet:** edema, headache, dizziness, liver problems and muscle pain

Medication	Generic Name (Brand Name)	Possible Cardio-protective Effects	Possible Side Effects
Fibrates	clofibrate (Atromid-S), fenofibrate (Lofibra, Tricor), gemfibrozil (Lopid)	Fibrates reduce triglycerides and, to a lesser extent, increase HDLs. Lowers CRP, a measure of inflammation.	Gastrointestinal upset, liver problems
Niacin (Nicotinic Acid)	Brand names: Niacor, Niaspan	Niacin: Niacin is the most effective drug to raise HDL and also lower LDL cholesterol and triglycerides. Lowers CRP, a measure of inflammation.	Niacin: Facial flushing (red, itching, tingling skin), headache, blurred vision, upset stomach, vomiting, diarrhea, heartburn, bloating.

Medication	Generic Name (Brand Name)	Possible Cardio-protective Effects	Possible Side Effects
Diuretics (thiazide diuretics)	chlorthalidone (Hygroton, Thalitone); hydrochlorothiazide (Carozide, Diaqua, Ezide, Hydro Par, HydroDIRURIL, Loqua, Micorzide, Oretic)	Otherwise known as prescription water pills, diuretics reduce blood pressure and swelling by decreasing the amount of water in the body by increasing the amount of salt and water lost through the urine.	Dizziness, tingling or numbness, excessive urination, muscle weakness or cramps, nausea or decreased appetite, abdominal pain, impotence, kidney problems, low potassium levels
Statins	atorvastatin (Lipitor), fluvastatin (Lescol), lovastatin (Altocor, Mevacor), pravastatin (Pravachol), rosuvastatin (Crestor), simvastatin (Zocor)	Statins are most effective for lowering LDL ("bad") cholesterol and modestly raising HDL cholesterol and may lower triglycerides. They also lower CRP, a measure of inflammation.	Liver and muscle toxicity (uncommon), constipation, headache, nausea
Warfarin	Brand names: Coumadin, Miradon	An anticoagulant (blood thinner), warfarin reduces the formation of blood clots. It's recommended for those who need a blood thinner but can't take aspirin.	Abdominal or stomach pain, back pain or backache, blurred vision, chest pain, constipation, diarrhea, dizziness, nausea, nervousness, numbness or tingling, bleeding

A NOTE FROM DR. LORI:
NIX OVER-THE-COUNTER NIACIN

If you're prescribed niacin, don't substitute dietary supplemental niacin, which is available over-the-counter, for the prescription version. Why not? Because vitamin supplements and OTCs aren't strictly regulated by the FDA like prescription medications are, over-the-counter niacin may not contain the stated amount of niacin (a B vitamin). It could also possess contaminants, such as lead or other heavy metals. Some brands of over-the-counter niacin have also been shown to cause serious liver damage.

Helpful Ways to Remember Your CVD Meds

According to the National Council on Patient Information and Education, about 50 percent of the two billion prescriptions filled each year aren't taken correctly. Think medication mistakes are essentially a problem of the elderly? Think again.

In a number of studies, it has been shown that those who are the most noncompliant with taking medication are middle-aged adults. Why? It seems that compared to the elderly, middle-aged adults tend to lead more hectic, less structured lives, which can be disruptive to routine behaviors, such as taking medication regularly.

Taking medication as prescribed is important to properly manage your health and your CVD risk. According to the Association of Poison Control Centers in Washington, DC, there were roughly sixty thousand cases in the United States in 2001 involving people who took, or were given, a medication dosage twice. And research on medication noncompliance has shown that a common reason cited by patients for not taking their medication as prescribed is they "just forgot." Skipping a dose because you can't remember if you've taken your medicine already can also jeopardize your health. While there are devices on the market that can help you stay organized, you'll need to experiment with what works for you. Pills come in all shapes and sizes, and they may be dispensed at all different times of the day in different quantities, so it's tough to come up with a one-size-fits-all solution. But here are some suggestions for personalizing your pill-taking routine so that taking the right medication at the right time becomes automatic.

Problem: You have more than two medications to manage.

Solution: Ask your doctor if there are ways to simplify your drug regimen to improve compliance, such as taking your medication once a day or even taking combination pills. Sometimes combination medications are more expensive, but not when you consider that it's even more costly to have a heart attack because you didn't take your blood pressure or cholesterol medication regularly!

You might also get a pill organizer—a compartmentalized container with multiple bins, which can be as simple as a small tackle box. (Be sure to buy one that locks if you have small children in the house.) Pill organizers are available in pharmacies and online; *www.medportinc.com* is a good place to start.

One of my patients, Sharon, a fifty-five-year-old public relations representative who has high cholesterol and high blood pressure, has found her pill organizers to be a sanity saver. Sharon's system: When she gets her prescriptions filled, she empties the bottles into a special vitamin/medication dispenser (a UV-filtering bottle with six separate compartments). Then every weekend, from her dispenser, Sharon fills two plastic seven-day compartmentalized organizers, one for morning and the other for evening, with the pills she's going to take the following week.

"Every morning during the week, I empty out one day's worth of pills from my morning organizer into another plastic box I carry in my purse, so I can take my pills when I get to work," she says. She also takes her nighttime medications from her night organizer. "Without this system, I wouldn't take my medication correctly," Sharon says.

Besides housing multiple medications, a compartmentalized organizer can be useful for keeping track of the medications you've already taken. Did you take your pill, or just think about taking your pill? That's a common dilemma with behavior you do every day, such as pill taking. If you're not careful, you can skip dosages or take a double dose—a no-no. By using a pill organizer such as a plastic, compartmentalized bin, however, you can simply check to see if the targeted pill is missing from that day's bin. Still, if you use an organizer, be sure to label each bin first with the name of the medication and other relevant information from the bottle. Otherwise, you're apt to load the organizer incorrectly, which is a common error.

If you take only one or two medications and find an organizer overkill, pill bottles are available that change color or register the date when the last pill was taken. Check your local pharmacy or the Internet for what's on the market.

Problem: You typically forget to take your meds.

Solution: Develop cues that remind you—perhaps in addition to using an organizer. If you're at a computer all day, you could program it to beep when it's time to take your medication. If you're more mobile, consider investing in a sports wristwatch, which can be set to sound reminder alarms. Programming your Palm Pilot, if you have one, is also an excellent option because not only does it sound an alarm, it displays text messages, such as, "Take blood pressure medication now." You can also purchase pill bottles with caps that beep at certain times of the day.

If your problem is remembering to take your medication in the morning or at night, another solution is to train yourself to remember to do it by placing your medication in strategic locations. If you have orange juice every morning, for example, put your medications on the breakfast table, and consciously try to take your pills every morning when you drink your juice. After a few days, as soon as you drink your orange juice, you'll automatically reach for your pill bottle. It's a no-brainer. Some of my patients have found that placing their medications next to their toothbrushes in the bathroom works for them, especially when they're traveling.

Another effective option for when your life is busy and not in its usual routine is to envision what you'll be doing when you take your medication. If, for example, you need to take your next medication dose during a business lunch, imagine yourself sitting in the restaurant, taking a sip from your water glass and then reaching for your pill bottle. Then, several hours later, when you're actually sitting in the restaurant and taking a sip from your water glass, you'll be cued to take your medication.

Stick with Your Statin

If you are prescribed a statin drug it may be life-saving for you. The problem is that many patients don't fill their prescription regularly because they don't "feel" different or don't understand why they are taking it. If you are not adhering to your doctor's recommendations, sit down and have a heart to heart with him or her and learn why it's so important to take your medicine.

Your Medication Checklist

A surprisingly effective, low-tech option for staying organized is to make a checklist of all of your medications, like the one that follows. Include the dose, the time of day you need to take the drug, and what the drug does. Keep your list in a readily available place, such as your wallet or on your refrigerator. (Go ahead and make copies so you have a new sheet for every day of the week.) Just place a check mark in each box after you've taken your medication or cross it off, like you would an item on your to-do list.

Medication Checklist

Medication	Dose	Time to Take	Reason for taking
_____	_____	_____	_____
_____	_____	_____	_____
_____	_____	_____	_____
_____	_____	_____	_____
_____	_____	_____	_____

Avoiding Medication Mishaps

Beyond knowing the basics, such as what you're taking, what the drug is for and possible side effects, as well as developing a routine for taking your medication, I have a few more suggestions for dodging medication mistakes:

- Maintain a medication schedule and stick to it. Try to take your medications at the same time each day. This will help ensure that you don't forget them.
- Take your medication exactly as directed by your doctor.

Don't crush pills or mix them with food, for example, unless that's how you're instructed to take them. Don't take them at bedtime when you're supposed to take them in the morning. You get the idea.

- If you forget to take your medication, notify your doctor or follow the directions that come with the medication. Don't assume you should double your next dose to catch up, which can be dangerous.

- If you experience symptoms that feel out of the ordinary, contact your doctor.

- Be sure to tell your doctor if you're taking supplements or any other over-the-counter medications, including headache remedies, laxatives, sleep and motion sickness remedies, as well as any other prescription medication. These all may interact with your CVD medications.

- Don't take another person's prescribed medications. That can be unsafe and could also alter the effect of your current medications.

- Store your medication in a cool, dry, dark place in a room other than the bathroom. The moisture in the air there can cause medication to deteriorate.

- If you're traveling, take an extra supply of medication with you on the off chance you lose or misplace your regular supply. Also, bring along your physician's phone number just in case. And don't forget your health insurance card.

- If you have questions or concerns about your medications, take a few minutes to write them down and bring them the next time you visit your doctor or pharmacist. Preparedness is always a plus!

- Don't delay getting your prescriptions filled. Even going without them for a day or two may be risky.

Herbal Supplements: Buyer Beware

Speaking of over-the-counter therapies, many of my patients initially come to me asking about herbal supplements. Many perceive them as a benign alternative or more "natural" than prescription medication. In most cases, I suggest they don't take any herbal therapies or any supplements other than what I prescribe, which is nothing in most cases. They often counter with, "Well, what's the harm in taking say, hawthorn berry? It's sold over-the-counter. And I've heard it might be good for my blood pressure." I tell these patients that it's not as simple as saying we don't know if it works yet, but it might not hurt. On the contrary, based on the research that has been done on herbal supplements, some have the potential for serious side effects.

Ginseng, for example, may improve cardiac function, but it may also increase blood pressure. Kava may decrease anxiety, but it may also cause platelet dysfunction, and large doses may be toxic to the liver. Licorice may improve coughs as well as other respiratory ailments, but it may also cause high blood pressure, pulmonary edema and cardiomyopathy (a heart defect in the lower chambers of the heart). All told, if you're taking an herbal supplement, be sure to tell your doctor.

Unlike prescription drugs, herbal supplements aren't tightly regulated by the FDA. As a result, there's no standardization within the industry or rules to govern safety or effectiveness. The FDA, however, can pull herbal supplements off store shelves after the fact if consumer use proves them dangerous. That's what happened in April 2004 with products containing ephedra, also called ma huang, a natural source of ephedrine, which were promoted to aid weight loss, enhance sports performance and increase energy. The FDA determined that it was associated with adverse health effects, including heart attack and stroke. I gave a lecture for the

American College of Cardiology about alternative and complimentary medicine and suggested that herbal supplements should rarely be used ironically. A few days later, a famous sports figure died of a heart attack after taking ephedra, which has since been taken off the market.

More research needs to be done before herbal therapies become part of the standard of care. Even if a particular herbal therapy happens to be good for managing a CVD risk factor, such as high cholesterol or high blood pressure, it probably has multiple effects on the body. But only by doing high-quality, double-blind, placebo-controlled clinical trials can we know if the good outweighs the bad. In the meantime, we now have a long list of medications we know, through long-term studies, help prevent CVD. Place your faith in them.

Antioxidants for CVD Prevention?

Historically, as scientists, we've been surprised by things that didn't work that we were initially almost certain would help prevent CVD. That's a lesson, in fact, I learned early on. In the early 90s, when I was in the process of earning my Ph.D in epidemiology at Columbia University, a patient had come to me asking, "Will it help my heart if I take antioxidant vitamins?" That was a good question, and to answer it, I began looking at the research. At that time, there were few antioxidant studies involving patients with heart disease. As a result, antioxidant vitamins and CVD became the subject of my doctoral dissertation.

From the onset, it seemed that antioxidant supplements would help prevent LDL cholesterol from oxidizing, a molecular process that's a necessary step in the development of fatty buildup in the arteries. It made perfect sense. If oxidation leads to arterial buildup, then antioxidant supplements would negate that process. What ensued were years spent collecting data and running a small randomized controlled clinical trial of an antioxidant "cocktail," as I called it, which included vitamins E, C and beta-carotene, a form of vitamin A. In the study, I had three sets of patients: those with CVD taking a high-dose antioxidant cocktail, another CVD group taking a moderate-dose cocktail, and a third set on a placebo (no cocktail), the control. In the study, I compared the three groups after three months. Indeed, my results showed that antioxidant supplements did protect cholesterol from becoming oxidized, suggesting it might be good at preventing heart disease. In addition to my work, there are now literally hundreds of studies showing people who had high levels of antioxidants in their blood, ate diets rich in antioxidants or took antioxidant vitamins were less likely to have CVD. Sounds like a winner, right?

After gathering data into three hundred carefully written pages, I was ready to present or "defend" my dissertation in May 1996. But a few days before the big day, the results of two major randomized clinical trials were published that showed the opposite of my findings, that there was no benefit to taking antioxidant vitamins with regard to CVD risk, and that there could, in fact, be harm in some cases, including increased risk of bleeding-types of stroke and lung cancer in people who smoked and took antioxidant supplements. Since then, more studies have shown no benefit to antioxidant supplements and possible harm.

What happened? Well, the big difference with a major randomized control trial is that you avoid the problem of "selection bias," which likely played a role in the earlier studies, including mine. That is, people who choose to take supplements may have other characteristics or lifestyles that protect the heart, and researchers may have been fooled into thinking the antioxidant supplements played a stellar role. As much as we try to control for this problem in epidemiological studies, we simply can't do so perfectly. That's why large randomized control trials involving thousands of subjects are the main types of data used to set clinical guidelines.

From that experience, I developed a hard line about taking medication, over-the-counter and prescription. My motto: don't take anything until studies prove it works. I think that's a good approach for herbal therapy as well.

Many of my patients are shocked by this approach and have a hard time accepting it. They aren't alone. In a national study I conducted between 2000 and 2003, 64 percent of the 1,024 women surveyed said they think antioxidant vitamin supplements actually protect the heart, despite randomized control trials showing the opposite.

A NOTE FROM DR. LORI: GO NATURAL

Don't confuse the antioxidant vitamin *supplements* A, C and E with the vitamins A, C and E naturally found in food (produce and vegetable oils are an excellent source). Studies show that eating a diet rich in these vitamins may, indeed, be beneficial for the heart.

Plan for Success: Be Proactive

Talk to your doctor about the possibility of a preventive drug regimen. Specific questions are always better than general ones, such as, "Do I need a medication to lower my blood pressure and/or my cholesterol? What are my specific goals and how do I get there?"

Ultimately, your doctor may decide that you're not a candidate for medication, but because many patients who should be on therapy aren't, it's important to open the dialogue. And remember, whether or not you're put on drug therapy, you still need to follow a heart-healthy lifestyle, which includes a low-fat diet and moderate exercise for thirty minutes each day because those important steps protect the heart in many other ways and may help prevent major risk factors from developing.

Three Keys to Your Heart

Here are three key points I hope you'll take to heart from this chapter:

1. **If you're not reaching your CVD goals by modifying your lifestyle,** ask your doctor if you would benefit from drug therapy.

2. **To take your drugs as prescribed, establish a system.** Get a pill box, use a medication checklist, or program your computer or watch to beep at the appropriate times. Experiment to find what works for you to help you remember to take the right medication at the right time. In time, it should be second nature, not something out of the ordinary. This is important because you may need to take the medication long term.

3. **Don't take supplements or herbal therapies unless they're recommended by your doctor.** We have many prescription drugs available that have been shown to be beneficial for your heart while we wait for herbal research to solidify. If you need CVD medication, stick with what has been proven and what your doctor recommends.

Chapter

Living with CVD

*"Courage is resistance to fear,
mastery of fear—not absence of fear."*

—Mark Twain

If you or a loved one has been diagnosed with CVD after having a heart attack or other heart problem, here's good news: it's not a death sentence, nor necessarily a ticket to a vastly diminished quality of life. After you've been evaluated and treated and your heart has had a chance to heal, you can often live a completely normal, pain-free existence with the condition, and maybe even appreciate all you can do that much more. My father, who continued his career with the postal service after his heart attack at age fifty-three, is a prime example. Now in his seventies, he still plays golf and enjoys spending time with his grandchildren, including my active teenage sons. And let me tell you, keeping up with them is a workout!

However, compared to someone without the disease, those with established CVD are at a much greater risk for subsequent cardiac events—so good control of risk factors is especially important in patients with heart disease. Heart attack may also be

complicated by heart failure and electrical abnormalities of the
heart, including arrhythmias—such as ventricular tachycardia or
ventricular fibrillation. These irregular and dysfunctional heart
rhythms can lead to sudden cardiac arrest. (This is the reason why
many offices and airports now have defibrillators available to
shock the heart back into a normal rhythm.)

Once CVD is present, there is no cure. Unlike cancer patients in
remission, heart attack sufferers will always have CVD and usually
need to take medication, in addition to adopting a heart-healthy
lifestyle, to keep the disease from progressing. In rare cases of
extreme risk-factor control, some blockages in the heart can
regress, but they are almost never completely reversed.

The disease will change your life, as it should, because the
alternative—denial—can be fatal. As I remind my patients who've
had recent heart attacks, there's a lot they can do fairly soon. "Can
I still have sex?" they ask incredulously. "Yes," I tell them. "In fact,
it can be an important part of the healing process." Just to be sure,
though, it's good to check with your doctor first. Although many
men and women can resume their sex lives within a few weeks, the
physical recovery from surgery can take longer. You're usually
physically ready when you can walk around easily. If you have
chest pain during sex, have lost interest or are just plain worried
about it, talk with your doctor. That's another reason to select a
doctor with whom you feel comfortable.

"Can I run the New York City Marathon?" It's possible, and several of my patients have done such races after going through cardiac rehabilitation. One of my patients, Peter, had an angioplasty
last fall and is going through the loss of a loved one. He was diligent about exercise and rehab immediately following his procedure, but this winter he has lost a lot of ground because of the
time spent caring for his loved one. We agreed that a way to get
him back on track was to train for a marathon or short triathlon

and to boost his confidence, I said I'd come to the race or run alongside him.

Post–heart attack, you can still exercise at a high intensity and get your heart pumping, as long as you've been through the appropriate evaluations and your doctor gives you the go-ahead. But to prevent a recurrence and the need for another angioplasty, stent or other lifesaving cardiac procedure, you'll need to be extra vigilant about prevention. Without question, you'll need to quit if you smoke, exercise regularly, eat a heart-healthy diet, lose weight if you need to, monitor your blood pressure and cholesterol regularly, and control your condition with one or more drugs, such as aspirin therapy, a statin, beta-blocker and/or an ACE inhibitor.

That's a lot to think about, I know. But you're not on your own in this, and you shouldn't be. To help you get on the right track and stay there, it's important to go—or make sure your loved one goes—to cardiac rehabilitation after discharge from the hospital. If your doctor doesn't mention cardiac rehab, tell him or her you'd like to participate so you can be referred to the nearest program, or check with your health plan.

Cardiac rehab is a medically supervised program that takes place in a hospital or outpatient center. It has been shown that cardiac rehab can reduce the risk of a subsequent cardiac event by 25 percent, which is significant. That's why I'm such a strong proponent of it and recommend it for all of my cardiac patients, like Pamela, the forty-year-old mother of two who claimed she just didn't have time to attend. Pamela finally went, and I was proud when she said, "It was so worth it. Thanks for giving me that extra push." Need even more incentive? Cardiac rehab can also help speed your recovery, so you can get back on your feet faster. Unfortunately though, less than half of those eligible for cardiac rehab take advantage of it. If you're diagnosed with CVD, count yourself among them.

The Rehab Routine

Once you're on board with a cardiac rehab program, be prepared for some serious lifestyle changes, includint what I've been emphasizing throughout this book concerning diet, exercise, stress management and taking your medications as prescribed. In rehab, you'll receive counseling, so you can understand and manage your risk factors and troubleshoot any barriers you may have to adhering to the prevention recommendations. You'll also begin a structured exercise program using a treadmill, bike, rowing machine or walking/jogging track that's tailored to your needs. In the past, if you'd been diagnosed with heart disease, you might have been told to take it easy for the rest of your life. Exercise was for the fit, the healthy, not someone who, for example, had a heart attack. But we've changed our way of thinking.

We now know that exercise is one of the most underutilized health precautions that even those with chronic conditions can take. If you have established heart disease, for example, regular exercise can lower the risk of a second heart attack by reducing glucose intolerance, lowering triglyceride levels and blood pressure, and increasing HDL (the "good") cholesterol, the benefits of which are intensified if you also lose weight if you need to. By being physically active when you're in recovery, you also set in motion a process of conditioning and enhanced day-to-day function, so that carrying a bag of groceries or tying your shoes won't be such a big deal. Many of my patients tell me those small accomplishments can seem like major feats, at first. Cumulatively, however, they add up to big boosts in self-esteem and increasing independence.

Through a cardiac rehab program, you can learn what you should and shouldn't do and the signs to look for which may indicate that you're getting into trouble. With the support of cardiac rehab, you'll get answers to any questions you may have, such as when you can return to work and what, if any, medication side effects you might expect. You'll be monitored for a change in symptoms by a nurse or another health care professional and possibly begin strength training, if your doctor says you can. If you need to quit smoking, you may go to classes or get individual help for "kicking butt." As part of the comprehensive program, a nutritionist will also help you create a healthful eating plan and teach you techniques that can help you lose weight if you need to.

Managing the Fear Factor

Emotional support from a team of health care professionals, as well as other patients who've been through the same thing, is also a part of the rehab agenda. That's tremendously important. As I know from my patients, having heart disease can be stressful and scary, like any health crisis. It's common to feel vulnerable, not unlike how it might be to drive again after you've been in an accident—only it's not the icy road conditions or the other drivers you no longer trust, but your own heart. "It's the end of innocence for me," one patient told me, a forty-two-year-old teacher who couldn't shake off the feeling that another heart attack was ready to pounce, like a lion in the African underbrush. If you were hit with CVD seemingly out of the blue, it can be shocking to know that you're not invincible. "My husband now realizes he's not bulletproof and he's not taking it well," one patient's wife confessed.

It's common after diagnosis to feel depressed, angry or fearful, whether you're the one afflicted or a loved one, and these are risk factors for CVD in and of themselves. Psychosocial factors, including depression, anger and social isolation, have been associated with an increased risk of death from CVD among those with the condition. It is important to look for signs of these reactions and get help when needed.

After a heart attack, even ordinary aches and pains can rattle you to the core, not to mention those who love you, evoking a sense of panic. One of my patients was a man who momentarily dropped dead from a heart attack, but whose wife was able to resuscitate him with CPR. Although he was fortunate to be alive, his wife hovered in fear that she'd need to repeat her performance. "I'm glad I could do it, but I never want to do it again," she said, after bringing her husband into my office to determine if he was on the verge of another heart attack. I had to do a lot of counseling with that couple to help them understand when to be concerned. "While your life won't be the same as it was before you were diagnosed with CVD, you don't want to become a *cardiac cripple* either," I explained. This is not an uncommon phenomenon after a heart attack. Being overly concerned about every symptom, or living in constant fear of them, can become more debilitating than the heart attack itself. Wives especially, often being the health gatekeepers of the family, can fall prey. "I want to be proactive," many tell me. That's wonderful, but being too concerned is also a stressor that's not good for anybody. In fact, if you're the caregiver of someone with CVD, I urge you *not* to lose sight of following your own CVD prevention plan, which includes, as you know, taking time for yourself each day to decompress.

Indeed, a diagnosis of CVD will change the way you look at life, but you and those in your inner circle will need to learn how to carry on in a way that doesn't amplify anxiety levels. That's why it's important to have someone to talk with about how you're feeling if you've been diagnosed with CVD. Some cardiac rehab programs offer support groups of others with CVD who've been through something similar, which is what many of my patients tell me helped them the most. "Without going to cardiac rehab and talking with others who also had stents put in, I can't imagine that I'd be so optimistic about the future," relayed one fifty-five-year-old patient who had just opened her own business after a midlife career shift.

Cardio Connection

Heart disease is a family affair. For additional support beyond cardiac rehabilitation, the American Heart Association is affiliated with Mended Hearts, a nationwide patient support organization for those with heart disease and their families, as well as for medical professionals, which provides support and encouragement to CVD patients and their families. For more information about the Mended Hearts chapter in your area, log on to *www.mended hearts.org* or call the American Heart Association at 1-800-242-8721 and ask for Mended Hearts support. Another source of support, Womenheart (*www.womenheart.org*) is a national organization that focuses specifically on women with heart disease.

Sticking with It

Of course, rehab doesn't last forever. Three months is typically the norm. But once you've "graduated," and are feeling a little more like your old self again, it's especially important *not* to slack off or go back to your old routine. Consider the principles you learn in cardiac rehab as a way of life. You'll need to eat right, exercise daily, manage your stress level, take your medications as directed, and get your prescriptions filled and refilled promptly to prevent complications. To renew your commitment, review the Personal Contract for Heart-Smart Living in chapter 2, and sign on the dotted line.

You'll also need to see a primary care physician and/or a cardiologist at least once a year, so you can be monitored for new symptoms and control of your risk factors. And, as I always tell my patients, keep your appointment—even if you feel fine!

Plan for Success

National guidelines have been established to help patients with CVD prevent a recurrence (and to help prevent patients with diabetes from developing heart disease). Here's a checklist based on those recommendations I give out to my patients to help them stay on target. Because recommendations change as new science becomes available it is important to review with your doctor on a regular basis. For updated information visit our website at *www.hearthealthtimes.com*

Go ahead and post this checklist somewhere you'll see it often and share it with your partner in prevention, who supports your efforts to live heart smart.

ABCD's of Heart-Smart Living for Those with CVD and Diabetes

A is for:

Activity

❏ Maintain a minimum daily activity level, such as thirty to sixty minutes of brisk walking.

Angiotensin-Converting Enzyme (ACE) inhibitors

❏ Ask your doctor about taking an ACE inhibitor. It may be part of your new prevention plan, unless it's contraindicated or you can't tolerate it.

Angiotensin Receptor Blockers (ARBs)

❏ If you can't tolerate an ACE inhibitor and you have heart failure, talk with your doctor about taking an ARB.

Alcohol

❏ Limit alcohol to no more than one drink per day for women and no more than two drinks per day for men. This is the same recommendation I give to my patients without CVD.

Antiplatelets/Anticoagulants

❏ Talk to your doctor about taking a daily aspirin (75 to 162 milligrams). You may not be a candidate for aspirin therapy if it's contraindicated or not tolerated. Avoid the use of COX-2 inhibitors. Be cautious about over-the-counter non-steroidal anti-inflammatory medications, which may increase risk of cardiovascular events. You should also ask your doctor about taking clopidogrel or warfarin, both of which prevent excessive blood clotting, if you have a coronary stent or you've been hospitalized for angina and you can't take aspirin.

Aldosterone Blockade

❏ If you had a heart attack and have heart failure or diabetes, and your kidneys are functioning normally, ask your doctor about aldosterone blockade therapy, which may be beneficial.

B is for:

Beta-Blockers

❏ Ask your doctor about taking a beta-blocker. It's generally recommended for those who have had a heart attack or have ongoing symptoms of angina, unless contraindicated or not tolerated.

Blood Pressure

❏ Maintain a blood pressure of less than 140/90 (less than 130/80 if you have diabetes and/or kidney disease), and, ideally, achieve a blood pressure of less than 120/80.

Body Weight

❏ Maintain a BMI between 18.5 and 24.9 and a waist circumference of less than 35 inches (women) and less than 40 inches (men).

C is for:

Cardiac Rehabilitation

❏ Participate in a medically supervised program after hospitalization for heart disease.

Cessation of Cigarette Smoking/Secondhand Smoke

❏ If you smoke, stop completely.

❏ Avoid secondhand smoke.

Cholesterol

❏ Get your blood cholesterol checked as often as your doctor recommends.

Work to keep your:

❏ Total cholesterol at less than 200.

❏ LDL cholesterol at less than 100, and less than 70 may be even more beneficial.

❏ HDL cholesterol at greater than 50 (women), greater than 40 (men).

❏ Triglycerides at less than 150.

Cholesterol-Lowering Medication

❏ Ask your doctor about taking a cholesterol-lowering medication (statins preferred). Statins are recommended unless they're contraindicated or not tolerated. Ideally, you should use medication that lowers your LDL cholesterol at least 30 to 40 percent.

❏ Ask your doctor about taking fibrates or niacin if your triglycerides or HDL cholesterol are abnormal, unless contraindicated or not tolerated. And keep in mind that dietary supplemental niacin isn't a substitute for prescription niacin because it's not strictly regulated by the FDA like prescription medications are and may have serious side effects.

❏ Don't take antioxidant vitamin supplements (A, C and E). They may interfere with statin therapy and are not proven to lower heart disease risk.

D is for:

Depression

❏ Watch for signs of depression and seek treatment if necessary.

Diabetes

❏ Maintain an HbA1c level (a reflection of average blood sugar control for the past three months) at less than 7 percent and a fasting glucose at less than 100.

Diet

Keep your heart healthy one bite, one meal and snack at a time. Your goals:

❏ Keep the saturated fat in your diet at less than 7 percent of total calories; that's 15.5 grams of saturated fat in a 2,000 daily calorie diet, for example, for small or sedentary people and 23 grams of saturated fat for larger or more active individuals who need 3,000 calories per day.

❏ Consume a diet that provides no more than 30 percent of calories from fat; this limit translates into 67 grams of total fat for those on a 2,000-calorie daily diet and 100 grams of fat for individuals on a 3,000-calorie daily diet.

❏ Try to consume no more than 200 milligrams per day of cholesterol from food. Foods with dietary cholesterol come from animals. They include egg yolks, meat, poultry, fish, seafood and whole-milk dairy products.

❏ Eat five or more servings of fruits and vegetables a day.

❏ Limit sodium to less than 2,300 milligrams per day.

❏ Aim for a fiber intake of 20 grams or more per day.

❏ Go fishing at least twice a week. To increase your consumption of heart-protective omega-3 fatty acids, eat at least two fish meals weekly.

D is also for:

❏ Don't take hormone replacement therapy if you're a post-menopausal woman to lower your risk of CVD. Discuss with your doctor alternative ways to control menopausal symptoms.

Prevention Pays

The saying "An ounce of prevention is worth a pound of cure" applies even if you have established CVD. While it's true that the medical establishment can save lives by surgically opening up the arteries with angioplasty and stents, don't rely on medical intervention to bail you out. When it comes to keeping your heart healthy, prevention is a major part of the game plan, even when you have CVD.

When to Worry

Although you don't want to be a cardiac cripple, life after a heart attack often means staying finely attuned to any unusual discomfort and making a judgment call about whether it can be ignored, or if it merits a call to your doctor or 911. Is it your heart—or just a muscle ache, indigestion, heartburn or GERD (gastroesophogeal reflux disorder)? It can be tough to tell. Here's a rule of thumb I tell my patients about when to worry: generally, if it *is* your heart, the pain or discomfort you experience will be similar to the pain or discomfort you felt during your previous heart attack or hospitalizations.

The body tends to use the same communication signals, its own repeated sign language that the heart is in big trouble and in need of more oxygen or blood. For example, if pain radiated down your left arm when you had your heart attack, that's how your angina will typically feel if your heart is in jeopardy again, although it may be much less severe. If you experienced an atypical symptom during your heart attack, like the patient I mentioned who had a persistent headache, take heed. "That's your sign to give me a call," I told him. On the other hand, if your symptoms are unusual, and you're not certain what they mean, it's best to call your primary care physician. When in doubt, call.

That's not to say that you will definitely get the same signs you did the first time if you're having another heart attack. You never know. That's why I continue to review with my patients both the common and less-common signs of a heart attack.

Common Signs and Symptoms of Heart Disease

- **Chest discomfort or pain (angina).** Discomfort in the center of the chest or an uncomfortable pressure or pain that lasts for more than a few minutes, or goes away and comes back. Other symptoms include heaviness, tightness, pain, burning, pressure or squeezing, usually behind the breast bone. These symptoms might radiate down the left arm, jaw or back.
- **Shortness of breath.** The feeling that you can't catch your breath, usually accompanied by chest discomfort.
- **Discomfort in other parts of the body,** such as one or both arms, the back, neck, jaw, or stomach.
- **Other signs:** Breaking out in a cold sweat, nausea or light-headedness, dizziness, headache, unexplained fatigue, upset stomach, rapid heart rate, feeling of impending doom.

If you have heart disease, it is important to keep nitroglycerin on hand. If you experience symptoms, you should immediately stop what you're doing and rest. If the discomfort continues, you should put a nitroglycerin tablet under your tongue (it will tingle if it's fresh), and wait five minutes. If the discomfort remains after taking three doses five minutes apart, you should call 911 or your local emergency service. Do not drive yourself or a family member to the hospital. Remember, the sooner you get medical attention, the less likely you are to damage the heart muscle and the more likely you are to survive, and often therapy can be started by emergency medical technicians.

Trust Your Instincts

Over the years, I've heard so many fascinating accounts from patients who've gone to the emergency room and who've had their symptoms completely dismissed because they didn't "look" like a heart attack. They were too young, fit or female (a nod to the gender bias, which still exists, but we're working on it). The ones who fared well insisted they be evaluated. "My body's not right. These symptoms aren't right, and I'm not leaving until I have an explanation," one patient said. Bravo! Although there are perspectives on this: from feeling sure you're having a heart attack to being over-suspect that you might have one. Overall, to prevent CVD from progressing, it's important for us to know our bodies and the signs of a heart attack and to simply pay attention.

Three Keys to Your Heart

Here are three key points I hope you'll take to heart from this chapter:

1. **Cardiac rehab is key to recovery.** It's a lifesaving step that can reduce your risk of a second heart attack or other heart problem and help get your life back to a new normal.

2. **Consider joining a support group.** Whether you're the family member of the person afflicted or a heart attack victim yourself, talking with others who've been affected by CVD can be a tremendous relief. But it's not just the collective support. My patients tell me that when they're with others who have been through the same things, they don't have to worry about burdening or boring them with their health problems because they intrinsically "get it."

3. **Control of risk factors is critical.** Recent research shows that patients with heart disease who substantially lower their risk factors, including cholesterol and blood pressure, will live longer, have fewer recurrent heart attacks, and are less likely to need angioplasty or bypass surgery. Now that's what I call motivation to follow your doctor's orders and take your medication!

Chapter

10

When You Want to Give Up, Don't

*"No matter how far you have gone
down the wrong path, turn back."*
—Old Turkish proverb

Throughout this book, I've emphasized that changing your life to be heart healthy is a process, not an event, a journey, not a destination. Yet as you review and employ the components of the heart-healthy lifestyle I've outlined, for yourself personally and as your family's "heart keeper," I issue a warning: be prepared to be at the bottom of your family's agenda. Initially, your spouse or your parents may "yes" to you and then ignore your suggestions about the importance of exercise and diet. Your children may roll their eyes, as my patients tell me theirs do, at your suggestions about turning off the TV and going outside for a walk together or foregoing fast food. Expect everyone to be resistant at times and to not always welcome what you have to say. You, yourself, may be inspired one day, yet frustrated the next. No matter how important or confident we may appear, all of us experience an uphill battle at times.

When you're met with resistance or overcome with uncertainty, hang in there and keep up the good work! Remember the goal in preventive cardiology isn't just to increase your life span, but your "health span," so that you can enjoy a good quality of life for as long as possible. With that long-term objective in mind, I encourage you to stick to your heart-healthy plan, taking it one day at a time. And keep in mind that even though making lifestyle changes may not be easy, it certainly beats the alternative!

When I was young and would get frustrated that school or sports or balancing the two was too difficult, my father often tried to encourage me by saying, "Lori, just tell yourself, 'When it's too tough for everyone else, it's just right for me.'" While this helped me a lot at the time, it was those dark, quiet, alone times when there was no "everyone else" that I found it most useful, when I really needed to face my biggest opponent—myself.

Because I am familiar with the territory of self-doubt, and being the preventionist that I am, I started preparing my children early on to recognize and work through times when self-confidence flags. My all-time favorite bedtime story to read to my son Mike was *Oh, the Places You'll Go!*, which was Dr. Seuss's last book, published in 1990. I still read it to Mike on occasion when he faces a big competition or change in his life. I particularly love it because it's like the pep talk my dad gave me when I was anxious or fearful about navigating new waters. The gist of it is that when the going gets bumpy, you'll find yourself all alone and afraid to go on. As Dr. Suess described, "and when you're alone, there's a very good chance you'll meet things that scare you right out of your pants." Still, you must face your fears and believe in yourself. This will be critical as you continue adopting the basic changes in diet and exercise that can cause a dramatic drop in the risk for CVD, for yourself as well as for those in your life who are taking your lead.

The good Dr. Seuss knew that the key to success lies within, that whatever external barriers face us, whether it's a sedentary job or seemingly no time to prepare healthful meals, we must first overcome the internal ones and tell ourselves that, yes, we can do what it takes to make healthy lifestyle changes no matter what the obstacle. Once we do, it's just amazing what can happen and the ripple effect that can occur. The rewards of your resolve will become readily apparent as you and your family not only feel better knowing you're taking good care of yourselves, but because you actually feel more alive and energized. By employing the information and tools I've presented in this book, great things can happen.

Quick Review

With one American dying of CVD every thirty-three seconds, we still have a ways to go in the fight to prevent heart disease for both men and women. Here's a recap of what you can do to fight CVD from the helm of your own family.

- Heed your own wake-up call and realize that CVD can happen to you—and your loved ones. No one is immune. Awareness is key.

- Know the common and less-common signs of a heart attack and what to do if you suspect you or a loved one may be having one. For a refresher course, see chapter 1.

- See your doctor regularly to discover and keep tabs on your risk factors for heart disease and your goals for prevention—from losing weight if you need to and reducing your cholesterol, to monitoring your blood pressure and your blood glucose level, if applicable. And, of course, if you smoke, quit. See chapter 2.

- Know your numbers. These include blood pressure, cholesterol count, BMI and glucose level. To keep track of yours, see chapter 3.
- Monitor your mental health by developing stress management skills and getting treatment for depression, if you suspect you or a loved one is depressed. It's important for your heart health. See chapters 3 and 4.
- Cordon off time for yourself each day to decompress and heal your heart by spending time with others and acknowledging the kindness in the world through healthy tasks, such as writing thank-you notes. See chapter 4.
- Exercise for at least thirty minutes each day at an intensity that's at least equivalent to brisk walking. Your heart is a muscle and it wants a workout. See chapter 5.
- Eat a heart-healthy diet, one that's low in total and saturated fat and rich in high-quality carbohydrates, including fiber, whole grains, and fruits and vegetables, as well as fish and fish oils and low-fat dairy products. Eat with your heart in mind and keep heart-healthy foods around. See chapter 6.
- Be a good role model for your children by exemplifying heart-healthy eating habits, teaching them healthful ways to cook for themselves and exercising as a family. These habits will save their lives down the road. See chapters 5 and 6.
- Put your health at the top of your to-do list by resetting your priorities. Remember, to accomplish everything that's important to you, you need to be alive, which is why your health should be number one. See chapter 7.
- Take your medication as directed, and get your prescriptions refilled promptly. See chapter 8.
- If you have heart disease, there are proven therapies like cholesterol management, blood pressure control and aspirin, which can prevent more heart attacks, hospitalizations and

procedures and keep you around longer to be with your family.
- The power to change and overcome inertia and fear lies within.

Putting Women's Hearts on the National Agenda

Personal change can take as much perseverance as societal change, which is something I know firsthand. As a scientist and physician in the field of preventive cardiology, with a strong interest in women and heart disease, there were times throughout my career I was so scared that I didn't want to go on. I've now expanded my passion for CVD prevention to a family-centered approach, but initially, I focused primarily on women.

When I first began attending scientific conferences sponsored by the American Heart Association in the early 1990s, I noticed that in a room of three hundred or so, only two or three would be women. I began to wonder why more female physicians and scientists weren't turning out at these professional meetings on heart disease. After all, it's an equal opportunity disease, one that affects women as much as men. Yet heart disease in women wasn't even a whisper of a public health issue at the time.

Since my own practice had its share of female patients, I decided to find out why women weren't on the national CVD prevention radar as a public health issue. At my first spring meeting of the American Heart Association Council on Epidemiology and Prevention, I asked to be put on the business agenda as a "new item," which made my mentor, Dr. Tom Pearson, who has a wonderful sense of humor, chuckle. "That seems appropriate," he said. But it wasn't so funny when I addressed the group. "I'd like to have a luncheon for women to address issues about women and heart disease," I said, only to be met with deafening silence. I could see my colleagues shuffling in their seats, some even snickering. If there were tomatoes in the room, I think some would have been lobbed my way.

Finally, an older woman at the meeting spoke up. "What are a bunch of women going to accomplish sitting around having lunch?" she said, obviously insulted, as if I were suggesting holding a bake sale. I was taken aback at that reaction. After some debate, it was agreed, however, that if I could document the need to focus on women's issues, I could present it again to the executive committee at a later date. In truth, by "tabling" me, I think they were hoping I'd go away.

I decided the best way to substantiate interest among physicians and scientists regarding heart disease in women was to do a systematic survey of American Heart Association members. Our council, however, only agreed to let me do a mailing to the female members, which is when I met up with a significant glitch: the mailing labels the American Heart Association provided couldn't be electronically sorted by gender because, at the time, they didn't collect that kind of information. I had to sort the labels by hand, with assistance from my Swedish au pair who helped decipher the international names. Finally, a makeshift assembly line formed on my family room floor where I stuffed the surveys into envelopes and licked the stamps myself before sending them off into the big abyss.

"From a little spark may burst a mighty flame," wrote the philosopher Dante. It's a quote I use to encourage those with a humble idea. Who knows? Your idea might change mankind—or womankind. As it turned out, the survey garnered a 97 percent response. We absolutely need to focus on women, my colleagues resoundingly told me. So I returned to the leadership committee.

"A task force on women needs to be formed," I insisted, displaying the survey evidence.

Over the course of the next decade, history was made. Our committee wrote a scientific statement on cardiovascular disease in women, which became the foundation for the 1999 *Guide to Preventive Cardiology in Women*, later followed by the 2004 *Evidenced-Based Guidelines for Cardiovascular Disease Prevention in Women*, which was a major collaborative effort of two dozen professional, government and other organizations that I chaired. The guidelines, among the top health care stories in the media for 2004, were the centerpiece of the American Heart Association's Go Red for Women campaign—a national movement to raise awareness of heart disease in women.

I must admit there was some resistance initially to developing gender-specific guidelines, just as there was resistance to a task force on women with heart disease. There are still occasional concerns that too much emphasis and attention to heart disease in women will undermine the heart health of men. I have to disagree and share my hidden agenda. I believe that if women are better educated about their risk, and learn about the risk factors, signs and symptoms of heart disease, not only will they potentially save themselves, they'll improve the heart health of the men and children in their lives because the reality for many families is that the women are the primary "heart keepers." In general, they're the ones who make the doctor appointments, do the food shopping, cook the meals and plan family time. Of course, this isn't always the case, but, in my opinion, arming women with lifesaving strategies benefits the greater good.

Meanwhile, our task force also helped give female physicians greater leadership roles within the American Heart Association. We provided names of women and minorities qualified for leadership positions to the executive committee. Within a few years, a black female was chairperson (the second woman in the history of our American Heart Association Council). We also established a young investigator award in honor of Dr. Elizabeth Barret-Connor—the first female council chair and a pioneer in the field of CVD prevention—and started a mentorship program to help connect new doctors and scientists with more experienced members. Leave it to women to nurture their young!

By reading this book, whether you're male or female, you're in an excellent position to be a role model for living the good life, for being a drop of water that starts a ripple, or a spark that ignites a fire. It has to start with you. You can change yourself. You can positively impact others. You can change the world, one family member at a time. When you want a revolution, whether it's within a major public health organization or your own family, you need to persevere. Remember, amazing things can happen when you apply gentle, steady pressure.

Joining the Global Fight

"Charity begins at home, but should not end there," said the seventeenth-century English historian Thomas Fuller. If you're interested in extending your efforts to reduce the risk of CVD to society as a whole, there are plenty of opportunities outside of your family. By joining one or more of the organizations that exist to collectively fight CVD, your voice and actions will join others in a causal cacophony.

By being active in one or more of these organizations, you can collectively help raise awareness, instill policy change, and improve heart-disease treatment for both men and women, so we can close the gender gap and have equal access to preventive and medical care. Organizations that need you include:

- **The American Heart Association.** Consider joining a local chapter of the American Heart Association and becoming a member of its advocacy committee, which helps shape public policy issues and laws affecting health care and such things as patient access to cardiologists, diagnostic tests and treatments, cardiac rehab programs, and the rights of patients to appeal medical decisions and denials of coverage. For more information about how you can help make America heart healthy and smoke-free, log on to the American Heart Association's Web site (*www.americanheart.org*), and click on "Advocacy."

  The Go Red for Women campaign is the American Heart Association's national call for women to take charge of their heart health. (I serve on the leadership committee for this campaign.) It includes motivational and educational support. Enroll and you'll receive newsletters, e-cards and interactive tools to help you stay heart healthy. Your support of this groundbreaking movement will also help raise awareness of CVD among women. To join, log on to *www.americanheart.org* or call 1-888-MY-HEART (1-888-694-3278).

- **Boomer Coalition.** The Boomer Coalition, of which I'm a founding member, is an outspoken activist/educational organization that aims to stem the tide of unnecessary deaths which result from undiagnosed and untreated CVD. It creates events that inspire and empower baby boomers to take responsibility for their own heart health. For more information, log on to *www.boomercoalition.org*.

- **The Heart Truth.** This national campaign, sponsored by the National Heart, Lung, and Blood Institute (NHLBI) and partner organizations, aims to give women a personal and urgent wake-up call about their risk of heart disease. First Lady Laura Bush has been an extremely effective and devoted spokesperson for the campaigns. To get involved and spread The Heart

Truth in your community, log on to the Web site for the NHLBI at *www.nlhbi.nih.gov/health/hearttruth/material/index.htm*.

• **Sister to Sister: Everyone Has a Heart Foundation, Inc.** Founded in 2000, this advocacy organization, which I serve on as chief medical advisor, works to increase awareness about women's heart disease through other women. Through our National Woman's Heart Day campaign, our organization hopes that women will encourage their mothers, sisters, daughters, friends and coworkers to get screened for heart disease and learn about healthful lifestyles. Sister to Sister provides free heart-health screenings at health fairs in major cities across the country. For more information, log on to *www.sistertosister.org*.

• **WomenHeart: National Coalition for Women with Heart Disease.** This organization's mission is to help women with heart disease take charge of their heart health. You'll receive information on the latest heart health research, notice of seminars, retreats and conferences on heart health you can attend and participate in, and join a nationwide network of women heart disease patients who are working to improve heart disease treatment for women. For more information, contact *www.womenheart.org* or write to: WomenHeart: The National Coalition for Women with Heart Disease, 818 18th Street, N.W., Suite 730, Washington, DC 20006, Phone: 202-728-7199, fax: 202-728-7238, e-mail: *mail@womenheart.org*.

• **Society for Women's Health Research.** This organization's mission is to improve the health of women through research, education and advocacy. The society advocates increased funding for research, education and advocacy. The society advocates increased funding for research related to sex-based differences in prevention, diagnosis and treatment of disease, as well as promoting the inclusion as women in research studies to provide vital information about contemporary women's health issues. For more information log onto *www.womenshealthresearch.org.*

Because of the efforts of breast cancer survivors and activists, women with breast cancer can count on an outpouring of public support. It's my hope that CVD will garner just as much awareness among women and men. Fortunately, things are moving in that direction. Today, there's a greater readiness to acknowledge the huge toll that heart disease takes on society, and major efforts have been launched to encourage prevention and better treatment. But much more needs to be done in terms of awareness and prevention. Besides taking the advice in this book to heart, remember that heart disease guidelines are changing all the time. It's important to stay current. To continue your education and get the latest information about CVD prevention, I encourage you to visit our NewYork Preventive Health Prevention Card Program Web site at *www.hearthealthtimes.com.*

Three Keys to Your Heart

Like all journeys, this book must come to an end. But your quest for living the good life with a family-centered approach doesn't. In fact, I hope this is just the beginning for you. As you continue down the path to a healthy and fulfilling life, I hope you will keep three key messages from this book close to you. (There I go with the three again. I just can't help it—it's the triathlete in me.) It's hard to stop sharing with you the wonderful lessons I've learned from my patients, my family and my profession over the past twenty years. But as Walt Whitman said, "Manuscripts are never finished. They're merely abandoned." The three keys to your heart I want to leave with you are the following:

1. **Know It.** Knowledge about your heart, your family and your risk is power, and it's the first step in living the good life.
2. **Nurture It.** Take care of yourself and your heart. If you're lucky enough to be healthy, keep it that way. If you're not, you can alter your destiny through your daily choices. As Goethe said, "Things which matter most must never be at the mercy of things which matter least." None of us can afford not to nurture ourselves and put our health at the top of our agenda.
3. **Share It.** Lead by example, and your family will follow. Who you are is what you do, not what you say. Share who you are to influence your home in a positive way.

Remember, home is where the heart is. Make yours strong and lasting—and the world will be a better place—one heart and home at a time.

Appendix

Recipes for
Heart-Health Success

Following are a few of my family's favorite recipes. They're easy to make, delicious and good for the whole family. It's not a cookbook (yet), but it's a start.

Picante Pepper Chicken

I can make this chicken dish on a Sunday, stash it in the fridge and serve it a few days later to save time. But my sons love it so much, I have a tough time keeping it around very long. I often have to move it to the Monday or Tuesday slot!

1 tablespoon olive oil
1 large onion, peeled and finely diced
4 large cloves garlic, peeled and finely chopped
2 tablespoons capers
2 tablespoons lemon juice
½ cup artichoke hearts
½ cup white wine
2 picante peppers, finely chopped

½ teaspoon coarsely ground black pepper
½ cup ripe black olives
2 boneless, skinless chicken breasts (about 1 pound), cut into 4
   halves
Salt and pepper to taste
1 pound spaghetti, linguine or thin spaghetti, uncooked
Parmesan cheese

Heat oil in a large skillet over medium heat. Add the onion and garlic. Cook until the onion is lightly browned and tender, about six minutes. Stir in the capers, lemon juice, artichoke hearts, white wine, picante peppers, black pepper and olives. Add the chicken and sauté on both sides until opaque and cooked through, about four minutes per side. At this point, chicken and sauce mixture can be placed in an airtight container and refrigerated for several days.

On the day you plan to serve it, reheat the chicken and sauce mixture and cook pasta according to package directions. When pasta is done, drain it well and add to the chicken and sauce. If your week is really tight, you can also cook the pasta in advance and keep it in a separate airtight container. I usually cook it al dente because when I reheat it, it softens a bit more, and we like our pasta on the firm side. Transfer to a serving dish. Serves six (or two very hungry teenagers and two adults).

Nutrition Information per Serving:	
Calories	388
Total fat (g)	5
Saturated fat (g)	1
Fiber (g)	7
Sodium (mg)	349

Grandma M's Refrigerator Cake

My younger son, Mike, is a chocolate lover—like Mom! He'd have mint chocolate chip ice cream—his favorite—every night if he could. But because it's better to have ice cream less often, we needed a chocolate substitute that was lower in fat. Solution? Grandma M's Refrigerator Cake, which my mother-in-law makes every time we visit her. It's a recipe handed down to her from her mother-in-law from Italy. Mike absolutely loves it—and talked Grandma into teaching him how to make it. Now he whips up a batch himself so he can get his chocolate fix whenever he wants. We seem to always have a pan of the "cake" in our fridge. It's low in saturated fat and calories and an excellent source of calcium, a mother's dream dessert.

4 small boxes sugar-free cook and serve chocolate pudding mix
8 cups skim milk
24 graham crackers, crushed

Prepare chocolate pudding per package direction. Refrigerate the mixture until set, about two hours. You don't crush the graham crackers. You line them up like lasagna. You line the pan first with some pudding them cover the surface with row of graham crackers, then pour hot pudding on it to let it soak in, then gently layer more graham cracker then more hot pudding not to press too hard so you don't displace the pudding underneath. You do this just for three layers and it all depends on how big the pan is as to how many puddings, milks, and crackers you use. This recipe should serve your family for a week.

Nutrition Information per Serving	
Calories	180
Total fat (g)	2
Saturated fat (g)	1
Fiber (g)	1
Sodium (mg)	217

Pasta Fagoli

Pasta Fagoli was of the first simple dishes I taught my older son, Matthew, to make. Because it's filled with beans, which are high in soluble fiber and low in fat, it's great for your heart. Plus, it's quick and a great energy dish before triathlons. Matthew can now make it on his own. It warms my heart to know he has cooking skills he can use for years to come. Bon appétit!

1 16-ounce can white cannellini beans
1 15-ounce can Italian-style stewed tomatoes
1 14-ounce can low-sodium chicken broth
½ cup small pasta shells, uncooked

In medium saucepan, combine beans, tomatoes, chicken broth and pasta shells. Bring to a boil; reduce heat and simmer, covered until pasta is cooked, about ten minutes. Serve with grated Parmesan cheese. Makes six ½-cup servings.

Nutrition Information per Serving	
Calories	215
Total fat (g)	<1
Saturated fat (g)	<1
Fiber (g)	8
Sodium (mg)	560

Old-Fashioned Chicken Noodle Soup

I like to make this extra-flavorful chicken soup even lower in fat by refrigerating it for a day before we eat it. Before warming it up, just skim the fat that rises and congeals on the top then discard.

1 onion, chopped
3 carrots, sliced
2 stalks celery, sliced
1 parsnip, chopped
1 whole chicken, washed
1 bunch Italian parsley
1 bunch fresh dill
1 cup spinach egg noodles

In a 10-quart soup pot, combine all ingredients except noodles. Cover with water until pot is two-thirds full. Bring to a simmer and cook for one hour. Remove chicken from soup and let cool. Remove meat from bones and shred; discard skin. Return meat to pot and stir in noodles. Return to simmer and cook for another twenty minutes. Serves four.

Nutrition Information per Serving	
Calories	325
Total fat (g)	9
Saturated fat (g)	2
Fiber (g)	6
Sodium (mg)	140

Low-Fat Fettuccine Alfredo with Asparagus

1 pound whole-wheat pasta, uncooked
1 cup evaporated skim milk
½ cup grated Parmesan cheese
½ cup chopped fresh parsley
¼ teaspoon fresh ground black pepper
16 asparagus spears, steamed and sliced into 1-inch pieces
Salt

Prepare pasta according to package directions; drain. Meanwhile, in a large saucepan, bring the evaporated skim milk to a simmer over moderate heat. Stir in the Parmesan cheese, parsley and pepper. When the cheese is melted and the sauce is thick and creamy, stir in the asparagus and pour mixture over cooked pasta. Season to taste with salt. Serve with Grilled Veal Chops (recipe follows). Serves four.

Nutrition Information per Serving	
Calories	535
Total fat (g)	5
Saturated fat (g)	2
Fiber (g)	4
Sodium (mg)	273

Grilled Veal Chops

2 teaspoons extra virgin olive oil
4 veal chops
Freshly ground black pepper

Lightly coat each veal chop with olive oil on both sides and sprinkle with black pepper. Grill or broil to your preference. When the veal chop is cooked, remove from heat. Serves four.

Nutrition Information per Serving	
Calories	225
Total fat (g)	14
Saturated fat (g)	5
Fiber (g)	0
Sodium (mg)	106

About the Author

Lori Mosca, MD, PhD is Director of Preventive Cardiology at NewYork-Presbyterian Hospital, where she runs a breakthrough program that teaches preventive lifestyle choices to at-risk families. She is Associate Professor of Medicine at Columbia University, Chair of the American Heart Association (AHA) Council on Epidemiology and Prevention, and President of the American Society for Preventive Cardiology, two leading professional organizations in heart disease prevention. She chaired the expert panel that wrote the national heart disease prevention guidelines for women and is Chief Medical Advisor for the Sister to Sister: Everyone Has a Heart Foundation. Dr. Mosca recently served on the AHA National Board of Directors and is a media spokesperson. She has received research career awards from the AHA and National Institutes of Health.

Dr. Mosca is the mother of two boys and wife of a pediatric heart surgeon. Her family cooks together, studies together and exercises together in pursuit of a happy and healthy lifestyle. A dedicated triathlete, she is a Hawaii Ironman finisher and continues to compete in triathlons with her older son (pictured above). Dr. Mosca continues to see patients to discuss their personal and family heart health.